Allied Health Professions – Essential Guides

Developing the Allied Health Professional

Edited by

Robert Jones

and

Fiona Jenkins

Series Foreword by
Penny Humphris

Foreword by
Professor Bernard Crump

Radcliffe Publishing
Oxford • Seattle

Radcliffe Publishing Ltd
18 Marcham Road
Abingdon
Oxon OX14 1AA
United Kingdom

www.radcliffe-oxford.com
Electronic catalogue and worldwide online ordering facility.

British Library Cataloguing in Publication Data

A catalogue record for this book is available from the British Library.

ISBN-10 1 85775 707 6
ISBN-13 978 185775 707 1

Typeset by Anne Joshua & Associates, Oxford
Printed and bound by TJ International Ltd, Padstow, Cornwall

Contents

List of figures

List of tables

List of boxes

Series foreword

The NHS, the biggest organisation in the UK and reputedly the third largest in the world, is undergoing massive transformation. We know that effective leadership is essential if the health service is to achieve continuous improvement in the services it offers. It needs people from all types of backgrounds – clinical and managerial – to step up and take on leadership roles to shape the future of health improvement and healthcare delivery.

Leaders are needed at every level of the health service. The concept of leadership only coming from the top and being defined by position and title is now out of date. It is much more about ways of thinking and behaving and individuals seeing themselves as having the potential to make a real difference for patients. Effective leadership is about working in partnerships and teams to develop a vision for the future, set the direction, influence those whose input is needed and deliver results – a high quality, safe, timely and accessible health service for all.

Allied health professionals operate in every setting in which healthcare is delivered. You have unparalleled opportunities to help patients to lead their own care and to see how services to patients, clients and carers can be improved across entire patient pathways, crossing traditional professional and organisational boundaries to improve patients' experiences. You have the potential to make a difference by leading improvement and managing services and resources well.

There are already many outstanding leaders in the NHS in the allied health professions making a real difference to services. Two of them had the vision for this series of books and have worked with formidable energy and commitment to make them a reality. Robert and Fiona have both made a considerable investment in their own professional and personal development and delivered substantial improvements in the services for which they are responsible. They have increased their awareness, skills and knowledge and taken on leadership roles, putting into practice many of their ideas and learning. They have worked tirelessly to spread their learning and skilfully persuaded a great many academics and practitioners to contribute to these books to provide a rich collection of theories, tools, techniques and insights to help you.

This series of books has been written to encourage and support many more of you to embark on or to continue your development, to enhance your leadership and management skills, knowledge and experience and to give you confidence to take on new roles and responsibilities. I am sure that many of you who have not previously considered yourselves as leaders will, when you have read these books, reconsider your roles and potential and take the next steps on your journeys.

Penny Humphris
Director of the NHS Leadership Centre
August 2006

Foreword

The engagement of clinicians in leading health services is of fundamental importance. Somewhat later than in many other countries, we are taking steps to ensure that we support and develop the skills and capabilities of clinical professionals for this aspect of their contribution.

Of course, many clinicians, including the contributors to this book, have taken the initiative in their own development and that of their professional colleagues. I very much welcome this book with its practical advice and engaging approach to this important series of topics. I am sure that it will find a receptive audience amongst the practitioners of the Allied Health Professions and beyond.

Professor Bernard Crump
Chief Executive Officer
NHS Institute for Innovation and Improvement
August 2006

Preface

There is a wide literature available on the theory and practice of management and leadership. However, to date there has not been a specific publication on management, leadership and development in the Allied Health Professions. With so many fundamental and radical changes and upheavals taking place at such a rapid pace in the National Health Service (NHS) at present, we believe it is the right time for a series of books in this field. Our series *Allied Health Professions – Essential Guides* – of which this is the second book – is intended for Allied Health Professions managers and aspiring managers, leaders, clinicians, researchers, educators and students and also for non-AHP registrants within the remit of the Health Professions Council. The series will also be valuable and of interest for doctors, nurses, pharmacists, optometrists, other professionals working in management and leadership roles and general managers within the NHS.

The books are set in the context of structural, organisational and management changes within the NHS and wider health and social care settings today, encompassing theory and practice and the many changes, policy and practice developments, innovations and new ways of working. All of these and other issues are discussed and set in the context of the NHS in the 21st century and Allied Health Professionals within it.

All of the contributors to this volume *Developing the Allied Health Professional* have recognised expertise nationally and internationally and are widely experienced in their fields. The text is not a continuous narrative, but a collection of subjects closely related and linked into the whole; we have not attempted to adjust the style of individual authors. Although each chapter stands alone in its own right, there are major themes which bring the different aspects together. We would like to thank all of the contributors for sharing their knowledge, expertise and experience. It has been a great privilege to work in close collaboration with them.

AHPs must be proactive and responsive to the many changes taking place and where possible to see the upheavals as opportunities, transforming them into positive steps towards the improvement of our services. There is no 'best, right or only one way' of developing the professional; our aim, and that of all our contributors, has been to indicate various approaches and provide an in-depth and wide range of information, which we believe will enhance the evidence base, knowledge, understanding and skills to support managers, leaders and clinicians to manage and lead their own development and the development of their staff and their services sensitively, effectively and efficiently and by so doing provide the best quality service possible for our patients and service users.

Robert Jones and Fiona Jenkins
August 2006

About the editors

Dr Robert Jones PhD, MPhil, BA, FCSP, Grad Dip Phys, MHSM, MMACP.
Head of Therapy Services, East Sussex Hospitals NHS Trust; Physiotherapy
Registrant Member of the Health Professions Council 2001–2006.

Robert is a Senior Manager and Head of Therapy Services in secondary and
primary care, with contracts in the independent sector, working at executive
board level. He has extensive experience in strategic, operational and change
management with a PhD in Management and MPhil in Social Policy and
Administration. Robert is a Fellow of the Chartered Society of Physiotherapy
and former CSP chair, vice president and council member. He completed a one-
year secondment to the Commission for Health Improvement as AHP consultant
and contributed to several DH working groups. He has detailed knowledge and
expertise in statutory and professional regulation and is a recent member of the
NHS Information Authority Project Board and National QAA Steering Group.
Robert has lectured at international and national levels on, for example, management, information management, service improvement and modernisation and he
has a wide range of publications in these areas. He is an external lecturer and
Honorary Fellow at the University of Brighton and a Governor of Moorfields Eye
Hospital NHS Foundation Trust.

Robert has led a wide range of service improvements and innovations, some of
which are national exemplars.

Fiona Jenkins MA (dist.), FCSP, Grad Dip Phys, MHSM, NEBS Dip (M), PGCO.
Head of Physiotherapy, South Devon Health Services, and Service Improvement
Lead.

Fiona manages and leads a physiotherapy service that covers acute care, primary
care and a care trust. Additionally, she holds a role of service improvement lead. A
Fellow, former council member and vice president of the Chartered Society of
Physiotherapy, Fiona has led a large number of multidisciplinary service improvement and modernisation projects across South Devon, one of which has attracted
national research funding and has been used by the DH as an exemplar. Her
current areas for service improvement include: physical and sensory disability,
Long Term Conditions National Service Framework, musculoskeletal and stroke
services redesign. She has successfully introduced several new and extended roles
within her large cross-organisational staff team. She has lectured both nationally
and internationally on a wide range of management topics. Her MA is in
management, with a particular interest in the management and organisation of
Allied Health Professions services. In 2004 Fiona received a Department of Health
award for innovative thinking. Fiona is currently undertaking research for a PhD
in management.

Both Fiona and Robert successfully completed the INSEAD NHS/Leadership
Centre Clinical Strategists' programme at the business school in Fontainebleau,

France. They have continued to work with INSEAD on the development of teaching cases for use on future MBA programmes. They were Modernisation Agency Associates and have worked collaboratively on service improvement, modernisation and joint national and international presentations and lectures.

List of contributors

Jonathan Burton MA, MB, ChB, MRCGP
Dr, Associate Director
Department of Postgraduate GP Education
London Deanery
Part-time GP Associate Director
Department of GP Education
London Deanery

Anne Candelin MA, Cert Ed (FE), DipCOT
Formerly Principal Lecturer
York St John College
School of Professional Health Studies

Sally Fowler-Davis MEd, DipCOT
Principal Lecturer
Post Graduate Programme and Business Development
York St John College

Margaret Gallagher MA, MILT, DipCOT
Lecturer in Occupational Therapy: Co-ordinator of Continuing Professional Development
Brunel University

Alan Gillies PhD, MA, MILT, MUKCHIP, Doctor Honoris Causa.
Professor in Information Management
University of Central Lancashire

Neil Jackson MB, BS, FRCGP, DRCOG, ILTM
Editor-in-chief of Work Based Learning in Primary Care
Postgraduate Dean for General Practice
Honorary Professor Medical Education
Barts and The London Hospital
Department of Postgraduate GP Education
London Deanery

Simon Loveday and Sheena Loveday MPhil, MA, BA
Directors, K2 Management Development Ltd
Cheltenham

Christine Lynam BSc (Hons), DipCOT
Community Mental Health Team
Selby and York PCT

Ann Moore PhD, FCSP, FMACP, Grad DipPhys, Cert Ed, DipTP, ILTM
Professor of Physiotherapy and Director of the Clinical Research Centre for Health
Professions
University of Brighton

Jane Morris MA, MCSP, PG Cert HE, ILTM
Principal Lecturer/Clinical Education Tutor
Physiotherapy Division
School of Health Professions
University of Brighton

Julia O'Sullivan MSc, BA (Hons)
Head of Continuing Professional Development
Chartered Society of Physiotherapy

Wendy M White BA (Hons), NVQL5, GradIPD
Assistant Director HR: Learning and Development
East Sussex Hospitals NHS Trust

List of abbreviations

ACE	Accreditation for Clinical Educators
AfC	Agenda for Change
AHP	Allied Health Profession(s)
AHPs	Allied Health Professional(s)
APPLE	Accreditation for Practice Placement Educators
BAPT	British Association for Psychological Type
CD	Compact Disc
CD ROM	Compact Disc Read Only Memory
CEO	Chief Executive Officer
COT	College of Occupational Therapists
CPD	Continuing Professional Development
CSP	Chartered Society of Physiotherapy
DGH	District General Hospital
DH	Department of Health
DoH	Department of Health
DHSS	Department of Health and Social Security
EBP	Evidence-Based Practice
ECDL	European Computer Driving Licence
e-learning	Electronic Learning
e-mail	Electronic Mail
EPR	Electronic Patient Record
GP	General Practitioner
HC	Health Circular
HCA	Healthcare Assistant
HEI	Higher Education Institution
HEFCE	Higher Education Funding Council for England
HMSO	Her Majesty's Stationery Office
HPC	Health Professions Council
HR	Human Resources
HTML	Hypertext Model Language
ILA	Individual Learning Account
IM&T	Information Management and Technology
IPR	Individual Performance Review
IT	Information Technology
KSF	Knowledge and Skills Framework
MBTI	Myers Briggs Type Indicator
MDT	Multidisciplinary Team
NHS	National Health Service
NICE	National Institute for Health and Clinical Excellence
NP-fIT	National Programme for Information Technology
NSF	National Service Framework

NVQ   National Vocational Qualification
OT   Occupational Therapy
PBC   Practice-Based Commissioning
PbR   Payment by Results
PCT   Primary Care Trust
PDP   Personal Development Plan
PPIMS   Physiotherapy Placement Integrated Management System
QAA   Quality Assurance Agency
SALT   Speech and Language Therapy
SCORM   Sharable Content Object Reference Model
SHA   Strategic Health Authority
SMART   Specific, Measurable, Achievable, Realistic, Timed
SS   Social Services
SSCs   Sector Skills Councils
SWOT   Strengths, Weaknesses, Opportunities, Threats

List of books in this series

Chapter 1

Continuing professional development

Julia O'Sullivan

Introduction

Continuing professional development (CPD) is a term that has become progressively more prominent in recent years within the healthcare sector. Familiarity with the term and awareness of both its meaning and its importance have gradually increased among health professionals as the demand for enhanced quality, efficacy and cost-effectiveness of service provision has grown.

This chapter outlines the concept of CPD and its underpinning principles, identifies the key issues and drivers, and describes some elements of the different perspectives of the Allied Health Professional bodies related to CPD. The chapter also highlights some of the systems and tools that can support CPD which managers and others can utilise within their working environments in order to help them to undertake effective CPD.

General concepts of CPD: what is it?

CPD is the learning in which professionals engage in the context of their working lives. There are several descriptions of CPD, most of which emphasise a planned and systematic process, recognising that, through increased professional performance, this should benefit individuals, organisations and wider society.[1] The most commonly used definition is that of Madden and Mitchell,[2] through their study of a range of professions:

> Continuing Professional Development is the maintenance and enhancement of the knowledge, expertise and competence of professionals throughout their careers according to a plan formulated with regard to the needs of the professional, the employer, the profession and society.

This description is summarised as that professionals:

- need to keep abreast of new developments in terms of knowledge, skills and technology to ensure continuing competence in their current job
- need to enhance their knowledge and skills to be able to initiate and respond to change in the working environment as additional roles may be demanded of them
- may develop personal and professional effectiveness and increasing job satisfaction.

The 1980s marked the emergence of continuing professional education when Houle[3] predicted that the growth of continuing education would outstrip pre-qualifying education. During this decade, many professions, largely outwith the health and social care environments – for example, engineering, law and accountancy – proposed systems of continuing education and a number of publications considered the conceptual aspects resulting in the term 'continuing professional development'.[4] Within the Allied Health Professions, most post-qualifying education and training was haphazard until the early 1990s when many of the professional bodies recognised the need for a strategy and structure for continuing education and adopted the term 'CPD'.

CPD describes the learning activities that are undertaken throughout an individual's working life and they are intended to maintain and enhance the performance of an individual in their working capacity. Individuals now work in environments which are changing constantly and these changes both generate and require a wealth of new or expanded knowledge, skills and information. It is becoming increasingly evident that it is difficult for initial professional education to equip the individual to either assimilate or develop this new information for the duration of their working lives. To keep abreast of such developments, there is growing pressure on individuals to develop their skills and knowledge through CPD.

The recognition of the need for CPD as part of the broader lifelong learning agenda is evident at governmental level. For example, the Green Paper *The Learning Age: a renaissance for new Britain*[5] identified the need for lifelong learning in order that Britain has a skilled, competent and adaptable workforce in order to compete globally and enhance economic competitiveness. This paper offers a comprehensive description of the need and the aims for lifelong learning:

> Lifelong learning should be for all aspects of life and meet a variety of needs and objectives. It should foster personal and collective develop-ment, stimulate achievement, encourage creativity, provide and enhance skills, contribute to the enlargement of knowledge itself, enhance cultural and leisure pursuits and underpin citizenship and independent living. This will require recognition of and support for a wide range of learning, undertaken in different locations, in various forms and through different routes.[6]

In the context of the Allied Health Professions, these have embraced the rationale for CPD and agreed a definition for CPD through the project 'Demonstrating Competence through CPD':

> . . . a wide range of learning activities through which professionals maintain and develop throughout their career to ensure that they retain their capacity to practise safely, effectively and legally within their evolving scope of practice.'[7]

Andragogical concepts supporting CPD

Andragogy is the study of adult learning theory. CPD is underpinned by andragogical concepts and those associated with reflective practice. These relationships are well documented in the literature. Examples include descriptions of the importance of adult learning theory and its application to practice.[2,8,9] Influential work on experiential learning,[10] learning styles[11] and reflective practice[12] has made a major contribution to understanding the way in which adults learn in the workplace and apply that learning to their practice.

An example of these concepts is offered by Kolb,[10] who argues that learning is a naturally occurring phenomenon and that the ability to learn is a proactive skill which allows us to influence and shape our learning environment. Kolb views experiential learning as a cycle involving action and reflection, theory and practice, and argues for a relationship between thinking and experience. The learning cycle is designed to bring about change and improvement[13] and has been adapted by many professional bodies to implement the CPD process in terms of identifying needs, planning action, implementation and review.

Kolb's learning cycle can be linked to the four learning styles identified by Honey and Mumford (*see* Figure 1.1):

- activist
- reflector
- theorist
- pragmatist.

In order to complete Kolb's cycle, ideally, individuals should balance across all four learning styles. This will also enable them to extract and articulate their learning and its impact on practice, be effective in their CPD and benefit from all types of learning opportunities. Honey and Mumford argue that individuals are different in their preferred style of learning and that preferences affect the way an individual learns from the learning opportunity. It is important that individuals recognise their preferred styles and also adopt strategies to develop others. Honey and Mumford also suggest that the prospective learning strategy, i.e. planned learning, is the most effective and best serves the aims of CPD, although the incidental and retrospective learning also has a value.

Reflective practice has been identified as a way of consciously analysing actions and decision-making processes, and developing theoretical insights based on experience and practice. Critical analysis and evaluation refocuses thinking on existing knowledge to generate new knowledge and ideas.[12,14]

The conscious development of reflective practice enables individuals to carry out routine actions quickly and efficiently as well as exercising professional judgements and decision making in new and uncertain situations.[8,15] There is a

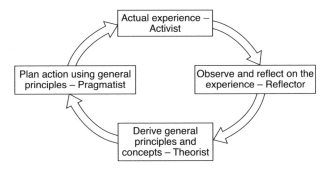

Figure 1.1 The relationship between the learning cycle and learning styles

fundamental link between reflective practice and learning, as the process is likely to alter the individual's perceptions and lead to changes in behaviour where appropriate. This facilitates the development of enhanced practice and improvement in quality. Reflective practice has been widely acknowledged in the health professions as a process to integrate learning and practice. Whilst it is recognised as an essential element of CPD amongst Allied Health Professionals, its vagueness as a concept and its complexity create barriers for some to implement it effectively. The required skills, and its application through techniques and processes, such as clinical supervision, resulting in both development of staff and improved quality,[16] can be addressed by providing Allied Health Professionals with appropriate structures and tools.

Although the importance of the theories underpinning the concept of CPD is recognised within the literature, there is little evidence to show that it is well understood by professionals themselves. It is possible that the application of this work is occurring subconsciously amongst practitioners but this needs to be made explicit to enable them to recognise and articulate their learning from practice and to become effective learners. This is an important element of CPD.

Principles underpinning CPD

The development of CPD as a planned, systematic, educational process is underpinned by a number of key principles.

1 The individual learner is responsible for managing and undertaking CPD activity, and the effective learner knows best what he/she needs to learn.
2 The learning process (*see* Figure 1.2) is continuous in a systematic cycle of analysis, action and review.
3 Learning objectives should be clear and should serve organisational needs and patient needs as well as individual goals.
4 The process is planned and based on identifiable outcomes of learning achieved.

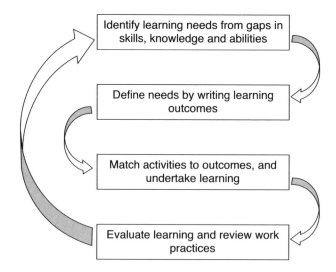

Figure 1.2 The CPD process

Models of CPD

Whilst there is agreement about the planned process of CPD and its rationale, there are different models of CPD which continue to create debate:

- input versus outcomes
- sanctions versus benefits and
- obligatory or mandatory.

Input-based model

An input-based model specifies how much CPD activity should be undertaken over a given period of time in terms of either hours spent or points collected and is linked to recognised learning activities. Whilst this is a straightforward way of measuring CPD, some may argue that it is also simplistic, with the focus on the activity itself rather than the learning gained and its impact on practice.

Outcomes-based model

An outcomes-based approach places more responsibility on the individual to ascertain their CPD needs and evaluate the learning, demonstrating how this has improved their professional performance. Within many professions, there has been a trend to move away from input-based quantitative CPD models to outcomes-based qualitative approaches to CPD. However, the measurement of outcomes still remains a challenge for many professional bodies. The Allied Health Professions piloted a CPD Outcomes Model in 2003 as a means of measuring CPD against six broad outcomes that encapsulate professional practice.[7] There is a continued commitment to an outcomes-based approach and the model provides a useful structure for CPD.

Sanctions and benefits models

Rapkins[18] identified two models of CPD policy and practice from Madden and Mitchell's research:[2] the sanctions model and the benefits model. The sanctions model includes compulsory monitored CPD for the purpose of updating technical knowledge and skill, and non-participation usually results in sanctions that can include loss of membership or chartered status. Arguments against this model focus on the lack of guarantee that compliance leads to the application of learning. The benefits model is voluntary and self-monitored and CPD is undertaken to update and broaden knowledge, skills and expertise. This model places emphasis on individual responsibility, professional autonomy, openness and flexibility but there is no guarantee that all professionals will take part.

Obligatory model

Later research has further distinguished the sanctions and benefits models into compulsory, obligatory, voluntary and mixed CPD.[19] Obligatory CPD is closely linked to the concept of professionalism as professionals are expected to undertake CPD which is self-monitored for both updating and development. There is, however, no checking of compliance. Many professional bodies assume this approach, linking it to codes of conduct. Compulsory or mandatory CPD involves 'policing' activity and is often adopted by regulatory bodies.

Examples of activities which can contribute to CPD

Definitions of CPD include reference to a range of learning activities, both formal and informal. A wide range of activities can legitimately contribute to an individual's CPD and there is an expectation that an individual's CPD will constitute a balance of planned formal learning and the incidental learning that takes place during the course of practice. However, there is no expectation that all of the activities are undertaken at any one time. Indeed, if that were the case, there would be no time to work with patients. It is recognised that the focus of CPD varies through different stages of an individual's career and therefore, the amount of CPD undertaken will fluctuate. In some stages, individuals will be consolidating their knowledge and skills and at other times may be striving to specialise or further the boundaries of knowledge and practice. The CPD activity should reflect these varying stages and the focus should be on the learning achieved and its impact on practice.

Some examples of learning activities are identified in Box 1.1.

Box 1.1 Examples of learning activities

- Attending meetings, e.g. clinical interest group
- Attendance at conferences and seminars
- Audit
- Certificated study e.g. Diploma, Degree, Higher Degree, Research Degree
- Clinical/professional supervision
- Discussion and networking
- In-service education programmes
- Learning agreements
- Learning from patients and from own experience of treatment
- Mentoring (staff and/or students)
- Post-qualification courses (including short courses provided by both in-house and external providers)
- Preparing and delivering teaching
- Reading and reviewing journals and research papers
- Secondment/work shadowing
- Self-supported or peer-supported study
- Significant incident analysis
- Supervising or teaching staff and students in the workplace
- Systematic reflection on practice
- Undertaking research and presentation of research papers
- Work-based learning
- Writing for journals

This list includes a range of both formal and informal activities and is not exhaustive.

Context: why the need for CPD?

The recognition that our early education does not equip us for all our working lives, coupled with a number of significant government developments, has contributed to the emphasis on CPD as a means of keeping abreast of new knowledge, techniques and developments in practice.

The government's agenda for health and social care provision seeks to improve people's health, improve quality of service, and invest to ensure appropriate modernisation. One major strategy to fulfil this agenda was the introduction of clinical governance which introduced corporate accountability for clinical performance, and mechanisms for improving performance in an environment where education, research and sharing good practice are valued through a culture of learning.[20] Other government initiatives, such as *The NHS Plan*[21-23] and *Meeting the Challenge*,[24] aim to encourage and drive staff development, through a co-ordinated approach and strategic CPD, in order to deliver high-quality services where NHS staff receive support from employers. The modernisation agenda for reform of the NHS includes the implementation of a Skills Escalator Strategy.[25] This is intended to offer a model career in the NHS, through a career framework[26] that represents growth and transitional change in order to meet patients' needs with effectiveness and efficiency. The Knowledge and Skills Framework[27] will be fundamental to moving through the skills escalator. The framework represents the staff development element of *Agenda for Change*[28] and will be a tool to focus and guide CPD.

These initiatives are being implemented in the NHS and affect Allied Health Professions working in this sector. Some have been adopted within private healthcare organisations and the social care sector. Regardless of where Allied Health Professionals work, they are expected to be responsible for the quality of their own clinical practice, and quality is closely aligned to clinical and cost-effectiveness and CPD. Maintaining quality in practice and improving patient care require individuals to keep up to date and develop clinical practice, highlighting the need for research, audit and evidence-based practice.

Alongside the increased demands for quality and accountability in the NHS have been the changes in statutory registration for all Allied Health Professions with the creation of the Health Professions Council (HPC) in 2001. The HPC is responsible for protecting the public, who use the services of HPC registrants, through setting standards of practice. The HPC will be requiring its registrants to undertake CPD in order to remain on the register and outlined its proposals for a CPD scheme which was submitted to the Privy Council in 2005.[29] Thus mandatory CPD will be effective from 2007 where registrants can be randomly audited and required to submit a profile of evidence of their CPD.

The implication of the government initiatives and the changes in statutory regulation for the professional bodies is that they have a responsibility to ensure that their members are demonstrably able to provide best practice. Thus, the professional bodies need to have a strategic policy and effective structure for CPD. Many professional bodies produce 'guides' to CPD and examples of good practice are frequently reported in professional journals.[30] The Allied Health Professional bodies all have CPD policies and a range of tools and systems. There are varying approaches to CPD between the bodies, with some adopting an obligatory, outcomes-based approach, e.g. the Chartered Society of Physiotherapy and

College of Occupational Therapists, and some adopting a mixture of outcomes and recommendations about the amount of time spent on CPD, e.g. the Society of Radiographers. All expect their members to undertake CPD. Some require evidence in order for their members to continue to practise, e.g. the Royal College of Speech and Language Therapists. Others have introduced a voluntary scheme for monitoring CPD, for example, the Association of Professional Music Therapists and the British Orthoptic Society. Despite the different approaches, the AHP project Demonstrating Competence through CPD identified a common base on the thinking on CPD and the nature of professional competence. Supporting members in demonstrating their competence is seen as a key role of all the professional bodies. The project was also important in bringing 14 professions together to work with a common outcomes framework. Since the completion of the project in 2003, the use of the profession-specific outcomes models has been variable. Some professional bodies have modified and continued to promote their outcomes model as a useful structure to plan, capture and evidence CPD.

CPD, professionalism and competence

The accepted purpose of CPD is to enhance the quality of performance received by, and to the benefit of, the client. However, CPD has been described as a contested and confused concept among professionals.[31,32]

In healthcare, the purpose of CPD is to enhance the quality of the outcome of patient care and patients should expect to receive treatment which is effective, based on sound evidence and up to date. Whether CPD can be related to demonstration of competence is debatable, as is the relationship between undertaking CPD and its impact on practice.[4,32–36]

A profession is autonomous, has a knowledge base and embraces adherence to ethics. [37,38] However, the responsibility for CPD lies with the individual as part of their professional role. Individual professionals need to demonstrate the ability to successfully engage in CPD in order to develop the knowledge base of the profession, practise autonomously and competently, and be accountable.[37–39]

The AHP project identified the following fundamental principles of professionalism:

- a motivation to deliver a service to others
- adherence to a moral and ethical code of practice
- striving for excellence, maintaining an awareness of limitations and scope of practice
- the empowerment of individuals and teams.

Competence is associated with knowledge and ensuring that practice is safe and effective. Eraut[40] argues that competence has a minimum of two dimensions, scope and quality. The first covers the particular roles, tasks and situations in which the individual is competent, while the second involves some judgement about the quality of that competence, ranging from novice to expert.

Allied Health Professionals are required to adhere to codes of professional conduct and are expected to undertake CPD. CPD is one of the responsibilities that is associated with professional autonomy. Likewise, competence is at the core of what it is to be a professional. The AHP project defined competence as having the following elements.

- Individuals have a responsibility to ensure the safety and efficacy of their practice.
- Individuals need to be able to think critically about what they do, rather than simply dealing with the routine or technical elements of their role.
- Individuals' competence does not exist in a vacuum, but is determined in part by their interactions with others and their ability to act, influence and respond appropriately in whatever contexts they practise.

The project sought to develop and evaluate an outcomes-based approach to demonstrating competence through CPD, through a common framework and profession-specific outcomes models. The key component of the project was the piloting of the models amongst Allied Health Professionals. The pilot exercise did not confirm explicitly that the models enable individuals to demonstrate their on-going competence through CPD. There is continuing discussion on whether the demonstration of professionalism rather than competence is a more appropriate goal.

Facilitatory and inhibitory factors affecting CPD

While the relationship between CPD and competence is difficult to define and the literature is inconclusive regarding the impact of CPD on practice, there is an inherent belief amongst Allied Health Professionals that CPD is a worthwhile process. Managers need to be aware of both the positive attitudes towards CPD and factors that facilitate CPD. Additionally, and perhaps more importantly, the inhibitory factors affecting individuals' ability to engage in effective CPD need to be highlighted.

Allied Health Professionals may accept the principles of CPD and have positive attitudes towards commitment to undertake CPD in principle but they need various forms of support to enable them to undertake it effectively. Managers have a responsibility to support their staff to enable them to enhance service delivery and patient care and to respond to service development. This can be done by introducing systems and structures, such as clinical supervision and journal clubs, and providing appropriate learning opportunities which will benefit the organisation, the team and the individual professional. Additionally, the working environment should be one that fosters and encourages growth through discussion, questioning and the use of research. Taking students on clinical placements requires all staff to contribute to their experience and can assist in the development of a learning culture. This is explored later in the chapter.

Managers need to understand the principles of CPD, recognising its integration into practice as well as understanding how their staff learn, both individually and collectively. There needs to be an overall strategy for CPD which might include, for example, protected time for activities, such as reflective practice or journal reading, as well as having a dedicated person responsible for CPD. The Chartered Society of Physiotherapy[41] has developed a framework for CPD to assist organisations and managers to implement best practice which includes 14 outcomes covering a wide range of issues to create optimal conditions for those working in a therapy service to undertake their CPD.

Some of the obstacles and motivation levels of healthcare professionals are described.[36,42–45] The main obstacles include the confusion of the funding sources and responsibility, and inequity of resource allocation for funding CPD, both between the healthcare professions and within the individual professions. Some study leave and funding is provided by employers for formal programmes and Allied Health Professionals are willing to pay some of their own costs, but many have difficulty in participating because of the cost and lack of appropriate opportunities.[36,43]

There is a distinction between CPD as an attitude of mind and an act of compliance. This distinction is important within the healthcare professions with the future statutory requirement for CPD and the professional bodies' approach that both ensures public safety and promotes professional excellence. Thus the motivation for CPD is influenced by personal factors, for example, career development and promotion, and external factors, such as fulfilment of statutory requirements.[36,44] However, the primary motivation is the innate desire to learn and develop to enhance professional performance, as well as increasing self-esteem and job satisfaction.[36,45] Henwood[36] included motivation as one of four factors and concluded that motivation was linked to individuals' job-related knowledge and skills goals and development rather than relying on a mandate for CPD. This can be related to the benefits and sanctions models of CPD.[2]

The role, demands and aspirations of Allied Health Professionals have led to conflicts associated with time and the guilt culture.[46] The guilt culture, connected with dedicating time for CPD, is due to the nature, management and organisation of the professions. There is a 'doing' culture rather than a 'thinking, reflecting and preparing' culture. Feelings of guilt do not sit comfortably with the increased demand for professional accountability, but the management nature of most of the Allied Health Professions is that all possible time should be devoted to patients. This is compounded by such issues as waiting lists, patient throughput targets and staff shortages. The guilt culture could be masking other barriers to undertaking effective CPD, such as the lack of skills to articulate work-based learning and to reflect on practice, and allocating time to non-treatment activities. Other identified barriers to undertaking CPD include family commitments, lack of library facilities and relevant journals, and lack of internet access.

Motivation, commitment and professional responsibility towards CPD are paramount but this needs to be balanced with realistic workloads, protected time and a culture that recognises learning and development as an integral part of patient care. There is a need to overcome the barriers in order to place CPD at the core of practice.

Support for CPD

The majority of the literature indicates that the responsibility for CPD should lie with the individual. However, effective CPD of any individual needs to be planned with, and supported by, employers and managers and guided strategically and in principle by professional bodies.

Organisational and managerial issues

Organisations are concerned with enhanced performance, competitiveness and cost-effectiveness and have a range of obligations if they are to provide the services to the public. The success of an organisation is, however, also dependent upon its ability to change and on the performance of its employees. Individual learning is at the heart of organisational change and development[47] and is central to the concept of the 'learning organisation'.[48] Senge[48] links the relationship between the individual and the organisation stating:

> Organisations learn only through individuals who learn. Individual learning does not guarantee organisational learning. But without it, no organisational learning occurs.

For any organisation, CPD must be managed on a continuing basis through the promotion of learning as an integral component of work and thus, introducing a culture of learning rather than occasional injections of 'training'. The learning organisation facilitates the learning of all employees and to be beneficial to both, it should have clear strategies to guide the integration between learning and work and appropriate resources to integrate them.

Healthcare is included in the governmental drive for economic competitiveness through its policy for the modernisation of the NHS.[49] Trusts, like other organisations, are subject to the influences of external drivers and are expected to provide a high-quality service with strategic direction. They are responsible for ensuring that staff have the right level of skills to deliver the service and to adapt or develop skills to meet new practices.[13] Managers within the trusts are expected to employ competent staff to deliver the service and to ensure that they continue to practise at a level of current approved practice highlighting the links between evidence-based practice, clinical effectiveness and cost-effectiveness. In addition, the public expects a qualified professional to be competent in his or her professional tasks and duties.[40] Thus, the organisation and the individual have responsibilities around CPD.

Creating a learning organisation

An effective learning environment is one where: questioning is encouraged, there is a forward-looking approach, practice is based on research, there is an awareness of professional development and individuals feel supported.[13] All individuals within an organisation have a role and responsibility to contribute to this environment which needs to have a framework to support this approach. The governmental drive for standards, quality and accountability has seen the introduction of, for example, National Occupational Standards and Investors in People, both of which promote education and training in organisations and can support CPD. Within the NHS, the emphasis on performance management has been driven by the introduction of league tables, pressures from the Patients' Charter and by the work of the Audit Commission.[50]

CPD should be linked to broader organisational learning and competitiveness and is likely to be fostered if organisations can see a return on investment.[51] Learning organisations are likely to attract active, ambitious learners who would like to foster and encourage learning environments to the benefit of all levels of the organisation. Systems have been introduced to enable and empower individuals to integrate learning and development with work. However, it is not the systems alone that will deliver staff development and a flourishing CPD environment. Key influencers within an organisation will determine its success and the level of support by senior and line managers is crucial.

Several authors[1,51,52] have stated the need for a deeper understanding of CPD, including workplace learning, by managers. Senior managers have the responsibility to promote CPD through strategic planning and practices to ensure that appropriate planning takes account of, for example, the impact of legal requirements, new technology, and changes in work practices.[53] They should encourage their managerial staff to plan learning and development to facilitate change. Within most organisations, the focus of control lies with line managers, who are responsible for developing staff to maintain and enhance performance. They usually authorise and agree development opportunities within a framework of general business activity and need appropriate training to do this as well as acquiring strategic awareness to manage their CPD responsibilities for both themselves and their staff.[52]

Systems associated with CPD

The ethos of an organisation can encourage and enable individuals to continuously learn and develop but this needs to be supported with systems and tools which have practical application. These systems need to be initiated from a management level with appropriate resources dedicated for training, implementation and evaluation.

Organisational systems have been established to develop organisational and staff performance from which objectives for the business and staff development should be identified. Within the context of healthcare and the NHS in particular, Edmonstone[54] argues that performance management implies the integration of a number of separate diverse initiatives at 'both conceptual and practical levels'. These include business planning, benchmarking, education and training, clinical audit, performance indicators, performance appraisal, all of which are the responsibility of different sections of NHS management.

Performance appraisal

Performance appraisal is one initiative that can be linked and aligned to CPD (see Chapter 7). Formal, systematic individual appraisal or performance review has been introduced in many organisations as a means of developing the competence and expertise of individuals in order to meet the organisation's objectives.[55] Its main functions are identifying training needs, setting objectives and targets, and providing feedback on performance.[56] There are, however, a number of concerns around performance appraisal, particularly the use of a system designed to measure managerial performance.[50,54] Within the NHS, the importance of performance appraisal in relation to CPD has been clearly stated with the requirement for all NHS staff to have a personal development plan as a result of the appraisal.[57] From 2006, an outcome of the Knowledge and Skills Framework development review will be the personal development plan. Linking CPD into appraisal and the development review process may tend to narrow the focus of individual development and potential within the current job as well as placing the onus on the individual, as often the developmental aspects of goal setting are ignored. However, it can provide a mechanism to help to structure and guide an individual's CPD.

Mentoring

Mentoring has its origins in advising and counselling[58] and can be either formal or informal. It is concerned with broad learning for longer-term development rather than short-term skill acquisition. Formal mentoring takes place in organisations with, for example, a 'buddy' system whereby individuals volunteer to either be a mentor or be mentored. The relationship is facilitative and a mentor is rarely the learner's line manager. Informal mentoring systems taking place outside the workplace can provide continuity, taking an overview of development. Mentoring can be an important aspect to support CPD as an experienced mentor can encourage and guide an individual to devise strategies to meet personal and professional growth. A mentor is concerned with supporting an individual, challenging ideas in discussion and shaping the way goals are achieved to plan for career development.[13,59] The importance of the personal qualities of the mentor is emphasised, as the mentor supports, enables and empowers the learner which is fundamental for the independent learner.

The real power of mentoring is the development of insights where connections are made between knowledge and personal experience.[60,61] Insights are difficult to define but examples include understanding of the values and behaviours of others, and how to work with others.

The benefits to the learner, the mentor and the organisation are identified in terms of enhanced skills, improved performance, job satisfaction and retention of staff. The potential pitfalls are also identified: lack of time, lack of skills, lack of management support. The significance of mentoring is that it can provide the link between off-the-job formal training and the embedding of new skills and knowledge through practice.[62] Mentoring can be a valuable support mechanism, focusing on professional development in the broadest context.

Clinical supervision

Clinical supervision can be a mechanism for mutual support and development of healthcare professionals. Clinical supervision is well established within some professions, for example, nursing and social work, but has only been more recently developed within the AHPs.[63] Clinical supervision is intended to increase the understanding of the professional issues through the implementation of an evidence-based approach to maintaining standards in practice. Its ultimate goal is to improve patient care.[64] It has been likened to a professional conversation designed to explore issues related to the effectiveness of professional practice and has been described by Butterworth[65] as:

> An exchange between practising professionals to enable the development of professional skills.

Clinical supervision assists practitioners to develop reflective and analytical skills. It encourages practitioners to examine their practice, identifying strengths and successes as well as weaknesses and mistakes.[64,66] It is a forum for disseminating good practice and, although there is little evidence to support its impact on direct patient care, it can impact on job satisfaction and morale.[67,68] The process can therefore support key aspects of CPD.

Successful implementation of clinical supervision is dependent on good management, clear organisational lines of accountability and adequate resources and should not be seen as a management-led initiative to control[66] or as a replacement for performance appraisal. There are different models of clinical supervision: one-to-one, peer, group and multidisciplinary supervision.[63] It can provide a formal system of guided reflection, consider organisational and managerial issues, define boundaries within teams, maintain professional standards and enable professional development. Although more evidence is needed to demonstrate its efficacy, the process is supported as part of the government's agenda on quality and can be seen to link with CPD.[24,57]

Peer review

Peer review, like clinical supervision, can be a system of support for CPD. It is focused on the evaluation of the clinical reasoning about a patient episode.[69] Individuals should select a peer who is similar in terms of grade, experience and knowledge. It can be a learning opportunity for both parties, enhancing clinical reasoning, professional judgement and reflective skills. There are different methods of peer review, for example, direct observation, documentation, questioning and discussion.[70,71] By analysing practice, practitioners can problem-solve and reason resulting in learning that can be applied in different situations and enhance the quality of care for patients.[70] Evidence of participation in a peer review process and the outcomes in relation to development and enhanced practice can be part of an individual's CPD.

Structured systems of professional support can be valuable processes within CPD. They enable individual professionals to discuss, question and challenge aspects of clinical practice and other managerial and organisational functions in a safe environment. Clear rules and procedures are agreed including confidentiality of elements of the process. Records of the systems can be public and documentation of learning outcomes, changes in practice and future learning needs can be kept in the individual's CPD portfolio.

Managers play a critical role in sustaining these support systems by enabling time to be taken to reflect and question practice. This needs to be embedded as an acceptable part of day-to-day practice. Many organisations have introduced these systems or have allocated dedicated time for CPD which is promoted by the professional bodies. There needs to be a culture of CPD where it is recognised and valued and meets the needs of both the individual and the service. Although the importance of CPD may be officially recognised, it can get compromised in practice in some organisations.[63,72,73]

Portfolio-keeping

A portfolio is a reflective and evaluative tool that enables individuals to collect evidence of their learning and development as well as planning future learning.[74] Many Allied Health Professional bodies, for example, the British Dietetic Association and the Society of Radiographers, expect their members to create and maintain a portfolio of their CPD. Some professional bodies have produced portfolios, guides or learning logs in both paper and electronic formats to assist their members to plan, record, reflect and evaluate their CPD. All provide guidance on how to compile a portfolio.

The key principle is that a portfolio should be a private, personal document owned by the individual. The fact that a portfolio is private indicates that portfolios are for personal use and are a source of information for evidence of professional development. Individuals may share some of the information but some reflections and analysis could be private and confidential to them. The individual has total control over the portfolio and decides what to include and how to structure it.

The benefits and practicalities of portfolio-keeping are well documented in the literature.[13,75–77] Keeping a portfolio may assist individuals to focus and organise their learning and to provide evidence of their CPD. In the process, they may develop learning strategies and skills which enable them to be more effective in their CPD. The benefits are highlighted in Box 1.2.

Box 1.2 Benefits of portfolio-keeping

- Focuses and organises learning
- Provides a structure for reflective practice
- Facilitates reflective practice
- Provides concrete examples of professional competence
- Assists in personal/professional/career development
- Encourages analytical thinking and provides evidence of learning rather than simply a description
- Encourages proactive, self-directed learning
- Active process brings about change in learner
- Making a written commitment to change makes action more likely
- Leads to connection of learning with day-to-day practice
- Improves practice

The portfolio is valuable as a source to extract relevant information to demonstrate changes or improvements in practice and achievements. There are increasing demands on healthcare professionals to provide evidence of their CPD as a means of demonstrating competence and performance. The evidence is submitted as a profile which Brown[74] defines as:

> . . . a collection of evidence that is selected from the personal portfolio for a particular purpose and for the attention of a particular audience.

The format of the profile will be determined by the organisation requiring the evidence and the information should be relevant, structured, up-to-date and succinct. Organisations requiring profiles include:

1 employers:
   – job applications
   – individual performance review (appraisal)
   – Knowledge and Skills Framework development review (NHS employers only)
2 higher education institutions:
   – accreditation for prior (experiential) learning (AP(E)L)
   – accreditation of clinical educators (ACE) jointly with the Chartered Society of Physiotherapy[78]
3 professional bodies:
   – mandatory schemes, e.g. Royal College of Speech and Language Therapists
   – voluntary CPD schemes, e.g. British Orthoptic Society

4   Health Professions Council:
   – re-registration requirements.

In summary, the portfolio is private and structured to suit the individual and is concerned with the processes of reflection, analysis and evaluation. In contrast, the profile is public, organised and concise with a focus on the outcome of achievements and can be compiled as evidence of the impact of learning on practice.

Summary

CPD is a complex idea which embraces a number of theoretical concepts. Effective CPD should enable professionals to develop the qualities of self-directed, proactive and independent learning. By developing these abilities, the individual should enhance their practice to the benefit of the patient and service provision. This development will occur through a planned and systematic process encompassing a range of activities focused on practice. This should enable Allied Health Professionals to assess their learning achievements, be more effective in their CPD and benefit patient care.

The formal requirements for CPD in the near future will compel Allied Health Professionals to submit evidence of their CPD. This will require both individuals and managers to have effective strategies for planning, structuring, implementing and evaluating CPD. There is a need to have appropriate structures, mechanisms and tools in place to support CPD and create a learning environment which values work-based learning, relevant programmes of study and portfolio-keeping.

The responsibility for CPD lies with the individual, employers, professional bodies, statutory bodies and government, all with different agendas. Can CPD be part of the internalised ethic of being a professional and also be externally posed? This is not clear-cut but the common outcome should be that CPD benefits the patient.

Editorial comment

CPD is underpinned by several topics covered in the first book of this series, *Managing and Leading in the Allied Health Professions*. Additional information can be found under the following headings:

- 'The evolution of the profession' (Chapter 3 – Robert Jones and Fiona Jenkins)
- 'Health Professions Council' (Chapter 9 – Norma Brook)
- 'The concept of clinical governance: 1998' (Chapter 10 – Amanda Squires).

References

1   Woodward I, editor. *CPD: issues in design and delivery*. London: Cassell; 1996.
2   Madden CA, Mitchell VA. *Professions, Standards and Competence: a survey of continuing education for the professions*. Bristol: University of Bristol; 1993.

3 Houle CO. *Continuing Learning in the Professions*. San Francisco: Jossey-Bass; 1980.
4 Cervero R. Continuing professional education in transition, 1981–2000. *International Journal of Lifelong Education*. 2001; **20**(1–2): 16–30.
5 Department of Education and Employment. *The Learning Age: a renaissance for a new Britain*. London HMSO; 1998.
6 NAGCELL. *Learning for the Twenty-first Century. First report of the National Advisory Group for Continuing Education and Lifelong Learning*. London: NAGCELL; 1997.
7 Department of Health. *Allied Health Professions Project: demonstrating competence through continuing professional development – final report*. London: Department of Health; 2003.
8 Aspland R. Workplace enquiry as a strategy for personal and organisational development. In: Woodward I, editor. *CPD: issues in design and delivery*. London: Cassell; 1996.
9 Lester S. Professional bodies, CPD and informal learning: the case of conservation. *Continuing Professional Development*. 1999; **2**(4). www.mcb.co.uk/virtual.
10 Kolb D. *Experiential Learning: experience as a source of learning and development*. New Jersey: Prentice Hall; 1984.
11 Honey P, Mumford A. *The Manual of Learning Styles*. Maidenhead, Berkshire: Peter Honey; 1992.
12 Schon D. *The Reflective Practitioner*. New York: Basic Books Inc, 1987.
13 Alsop A. *Continuing Professional Development: a guide for therapists*. Oxford: Blackwell Science; 2000.
14 Boud D, Keogh R, Walker D. *Reflection: turning experience into learning*. London: Kogan Page; 1985.
15 Eraut M. Schon. Shock: a case for reframing reflection-in-action. *Teachers and Teaching*. 1995; **1**: 9–22.
16 Cole M. Learning through reflective practice: a professional approach to effective continuing professional development among healthcare professionals. *Research in Post-Compulsory Education*. 2000; **5**(1) 23–38.
17 Chartered Society of Physiotherapy. *Developing a Portfolio: a guide for Chartered Society of Physiotherapy members*. London: Chartered Society of Physiotherapy; 2001.
18 Rapkins C. Best practice for continuing professional development: professional bodies facing the challenge. In: Woodward I, editor. *CPD: issues in design and delivery*. London: Cassell; 1996.
19 Friedman A, Durkin C, Hurran N. *Building a CPD Network on the Internet*. Bristol: Professional Associations Research Network; 1999.
20 Department of Health. *A First Class Service: quality in the new NHS*. London: Department of Health; 1998.
21 Department of Health. *The NHS Plan: a plan for investment, a plan for reform*. London: Department of Health; 2000.
22 Scottish Executive Health Department. *Our National Health. A Plan for Action, a Plan for Change*. Edinburgh: Scottish Executive Health Department; 2000.
23 National Assembly for Wales. *A Plan for the NHS with its Partners. Improving health in Wales*. Cardiff: National Assembly for Wales; 2001.
24 Department of Health. *Meeting the Challenge: a strategy for the Allied Health Professions*. London: Stationery Office; 2000.
25 Department of Health. *Introduction to the Skills Escalator*. 2004. Available at: http://www.dh.gov.uk/PolicyAndGuidance/HumanResourcesAndTraining/ModelEmployee/SkillsEscalatorArticle/fs/en?CONTENT_ID=4055527&chk=ZI7IKI (Accessed on 23 February 2005).
26 Department of Health. *A Career Framework for the NHS. Discussion Document – version 2*. London: Department of Health; 2004.
27 Department of Health. *The NHS Knowledge and Skills Framework and the Development Review Process*. London: Department of Health; 2004.

28 Department of Health. *Agenda for Change*. London: HMSO; 2004. Available at: www.dh.gov.uk/PolicyAndGuidance/HumanResourcesAndTraining/ModernisingPay/ AgendaForChange/fs/en (accessed 23 February 2005).

29 Health Professions Council. *Continuing Professional Development – Consultation Paper*. London: Health Professions Council; 2004.

30 Sadler-Smith E, Badger B. The HR practitioner's perspective on continuing professional development. *Human Resource Management Journal*. 1999; **8**(4): 66–75.

31 Friedman A, Davis K, Phillips ME. *Continuing Professional Development in the UK: attitudes*. PARN, Bristol; 2001.

32 Phillips M, Doheny S, Hearn C *et al*. *The Impact of Continuing Professional Development*. Bristol: University of Bristol; 2004.

33 Ferguson A. Evaluating the purpose and benefits of continuing education in nursing and the implications for the provision of continuing education for cancer nurses. *Journal of Advance Nursing*. 1994; **19**: 640–46.

34 McCormick G, Marshall E. Mandatory Continuing Professional Education: a review. *Australian Physiotherapy*. 1994; **40**(1) 17–22.

35 Powell A. *A Framework for Continuing Professional Development – A Feasibility Study – Final Report*. London: Chartered Society of Physiotherapy; 1997.

36 Henwood SM, Benwell MJ. Continuing Professional Development for Radiographers: a review of the literature. *Journal of Diagnostic Radiography and Imaging*. 1998; **1**: 17–25.

37 Higgs J. Physiotherapy, Professionalism and Self-directed Learning. *Journal of Singapore Physiotherapy Association*. 1993; **14**(1): 8–11.

38 Bossers A, Kernaghan J, Hodgins L *et al*. Defining and developing professionalism. *Canadian Journal of Occupational Therapy*. 1999; **66**(3): 116–21.

39 Haines PJ. Professionalization through CPD: is it realistic for achieving our goals? *British Journal of Therapy and Rehabilitation*. 1997; **4**(8): 428–47.

40 Eraut M. *Developing Professional Knowledge and Competence*. London: The Falmer Press; 1994.

41 Chartered Society of Physiotherapy. *Framework for the Creation of Successful Systems of CPD in Physiotherapy Services*. London: Chartered Society of Physiotherapy; 2003.

42 Cutts A, Johnson GR, Fielding SA. Rehabilitation engineering courses for rehabilitation professionals – an investigation of demands and requirements. *Clinical Rehabilitation*. 1994; **8**: 1–6.

43 Maxwell M. Continuing education in physiotherapy. *Medical Teacher*. 1995; **17**(2): 189–97.

44 Calpin Davies PJ. Purchasing post-qualifying professional education in the healthcare sector. *Journal of Nursing Management*. 1996; **4**: 133–41.

45 Laszlo H, Strettle RJ. Midwives' motivation for continuing education. *Nurse Education Today*. 1996; **16**: 363–7.

46 O'Sullivan J. Unlocking the workforce potential: is support for effective continuing professional development (CPD) the key? *Research in Post-Compulsory Education Issue*. 2003; **8**(1) 107–22.

47 Boulstridge B, Cooper N. Stimulating creative and critical energies in the process of organisational change and development. In: Woodward I, editor. *CPD: issues in design and delivery*. London: Cassell ; 1996.

48 Senge PM. *The Fifth Discipline Fieldbook: strategies and tools for building a learning organisation*. New York: Doubleday; 1994.

49 Department of Health. *The New NHS: modern, dependable*. London: Department of Health; 1997.

50 Redman T. *Performance Appraisal Effectiveness: evidence from the NHS*. School of Business and Management, University of Teesside, 1997.

51 Sandelands E. Emerging issues in Continuing Professional Development. *Continuing*

Professional Development. 1998. 1. http://openhouse.org.uk/virtual-university-press/cpd/.

52 Jones N, Robinson G. Do organizations manage continuing professional development? *Continuing Professional Development*. 1998. 1. http://openhouse.org.uk/virtual-university-press/cpd/.

53 Wood S, editor. *Continuous Development: the path to improved performance*. London: Institute of Personnel and Development; 1994.

54 Edmonstone J. Appraising the state of performance appraisal. *Health Manpower Management*. 1996; **22**(6): 9–13.

55 Fletcher C. *Appraisal: routes to improved performance*. London: Institute of Personnel and Development; 1993.

56 The Industrial Society. *Appraisal. Managing Best Practice* No 37. London: The Industrial Society; 1997.

57 Department of Health. *Continuing Professional Development: quality in the new NHS*. London: Department of Health; 1999.

58 Parsloe E. *The Manager as Coach and Mentor*. London: Institute of Personnel and Development; 1995.

59 Coles C. Approaching professional development. *Journal of Continuing Education in the Health Professions*. 1996; **16**: 152–8.

60 Mumford A. Sources for courses. *People Management*. 1998. **14 May**: 48–50.

61 Hale R. The Dynamics of Mentoring Relationships: towards an understanding of how mentoring supports learning. *Continuing Professional Development*. 1998. **3**. www.openhouse.org.uk/virtual-university-press/.

62 Chartered Society of Physiotherapy. *Mentoring*. CPD Information Paper No 35. London: Chartered Society of Physiotherapy; 2004.

63 Sellars J. Learning from Contemporary Practice: an explanation of clinical supervision in physiotherapy. *Learning in Health and Social Care*. 2004; **3**(2): 64–82.

64 Mattson M. Supervision under a magnifying glass: characteristics of physiotherapy unveiled. *Nordic Physiotherapy*. 1995; **2**(7 Supplement): 12–19.

65 Butterworth T. Clinical Supervision as an emerging idea in nursing. In: Butterworth T, Faugier J, Burnard P, editors. *Clinical Supervision and Mentorship in Nursing*. Cheltenham: Stanley Thornes Ltd; 1998.

66 Thomas S. Clinical Supervision. *Journal of Community Nursing*. 1995; **10**: 12–18.

67 Sloan G. Clinical Supervision: characteristics of a good supervisor. *Nursing Standard*. 1998; **12**(40): 42–6.

68 Cutcliffe JR, Epling M, Cassedy P *et al*. Ethical dilemmas in clinical supervision 1: need for guidelines. *British Journal of Nursing*. 1998; **7**(15): 920–23.

69 Chartered Society of Physiotherapy. *Standards of Physiotherapy Practice*. London: Chartered Society of Physiotherapy; 2005.

70 Slater DY, Cohn ES. Staff development through analysis of practice. *American Journal of Occupational Therapy*. 1991; **45**(11): 1038–44.

71 Hagedorn R. Clinical decision making in familiar cases: a model of the process and implications for practice. *British Journal of Occupational Therapy*. 1996; **59**(5): 217–22.

72 Brown A. Professionals under pressure: contextual influences on learning and development of radiographers in England. *Learning in Health and Social Care*. 2004; **3**(4): 213–22.

73 Chia SH, Harrison D, editors. *Tools for Continuing Professional Development*. Wiltshire: Quay Books; 2004.

74 Brown RA. *Portfolio Development and Profiling for Nurses*. Lancaster: Quay Books; 1992.

75 Hull C, Redfern L. *Profiles and Portfolios – A Guide for Nurses and Midwives*. Basingstoke: Macmillan; 1996.

76 O'Sullivan J. *Changing Patterns of CPD Activity: Evaluation of CPD Workshops*. Proceedings of the International Ottawa Conference on Medical Education, Barcelona, Spain; 2004.

77 Stewart S. The place of portfolios within continuing professional development. In: Chia SH, Harrison D, editors. *Tools for Continuing Professional Development.* Wiltshire: Quay Books; 2004.

78 Chartered Society of Physiotherapy. *Accreditation of Clinical Educators Scheme.* London: Chartered Society of Physiotherapy; 2004.

Chapter 2

Clinical supervision for postgraduate Allied Health Professions

Margaret Gallagher

There are challenging questions about how we nurture and promote good practice with novice practitioners and how we support progression for experienced staff. We can therefore be forgiven if we feel that we have been abandoned in the 'matrix' with little understanding of the complex mechanisms intrinsically involved in clinical supervision.

As a new manager some years ago, one of my first tasks was to commission and establish a formal supervision framework in the service. This laid out clear expectations of what supervision was and how it was to be conducted. The feedback from staff was generally positive. The process we used was a hierarchical approach, with staff supervised by their direct line manager. This had the merit of providing a formal and equitable process for all staff, both qualified and support staff. Training for staff in preparation for either giving or receiving supervision was not included in this approach as there was a naïve assumption that this could be done through existing skills and knowledge. The potential conflict within the staff/manager relationship was not addressed. In retrospect this approach was primarily a managerial tool for managing the service, with some consideration given to staff development. The main context was one of significant service change and to a limited degree this mechanism gave the service a framework through which we could communicate and support staff through the changes. It was not revolutionary but seen to be an effective tool to both recruit and retain staff.

The selection of appropriate clinical supervision frameworks is crucial to assist health professionals to increase their repertoire of practice, informing and empowering them to make effective decisions, and at the same time enabling them to experiment safely with their knowledge and understanding.

This chapter discusses the context and origins of supervision, the many definitions and perceptions, the purpose (and links to reflective practice), approaches to and evaluation of supervision. The chapter will also focus on evidence from the literature that provides not only guidance to clinical supervision but also an awareness of the potential tensions, so that managers may develop effective approaches to clinical supervision. It will also explore the void between our understanding of clinical supervision from pre-registration experience and our understanding of our therapeutic relationships with clients and patients. It is hoped that this chapter will facilitate progression and insight into the reader's process and practice, and explore ways of providing clinical supervision for staff currently supervised and for those future supervisees.

Seeking a balanced and manageable approach to delivering an effective clinical supervision framework is not an easy task. Clinical supervision requires us to be critical managers of our careers and development. Maintaining professional autonomy at the same time as responding to the Department of Health (DH) exhortations of good practice requires significant skill. The Health Professions Council and professional associations' requirements confirm the duties and professional responsibilities of healthcare professionals. For many, including the DH and our professional associations, the notion of clinical supervision has inherent merit, and is a beguiling, seductive notion when looking at the risks involved for organisations and individuals in delivering healthcare to clients and patients in the 21st century. However, the evidence from the literature regarding the efficacy of clinical supervision is ambiguous and conflicting and can leave the manager and practitioner confused. Being required to undertake clinical supervision does not necessarily connect with an intrinsic understanding of how complex and potentially demanding the process can be.

Context of clinical supervision

The UK government's drive to implement clinical supervision should be seen in the light of the need to manage the risk of poor or negligent practice, Bristol 2001[1] and Alder Hey 2001.[2] The current context of clinical supervision is delivered through the framework of clinical governance, which was introduced through *The New NHS: modern, dependable* in 1997,[3] and *A First Class Service: quality in the new NHS* in 1998.[4] Clinical governance was introduced as a quality assurance mechanism in healthcare to support professional development, reduce risk and as a performance management process. It has been defined as:

> A framework through which NHS organisations are accountable for continually improving the quality of their services and safeguarding high standards of care by creating an environment in which excellence in clinical care will flourish.[5]

Clinical governance requires clear lines of accountability and responsibility, for practitioners to deliver evidence-based practice and clinical effectiveness. Also the government drive for lifelong learning has been enshrined within both Department of Health initiatives and professional bodies,[6] supporting the concept of continuing professional development (CPD). All these elements are included within clinical supervision, with the aim of improving practice and reducing risks.

The creation of consultant therapists posts from *The NHS Plan*[7] and *Meeting the Challenge*[8] provided new opportunities and roles for therapists to strategically change both practice and the delivery of services. The role and potential contribution of clinical supervision in the development of these new roles need to be explored.

The implementation of *Agenda for Change*,[9] the modernisation of the NHS pay systems, is effectively changing career pathways in the NHS. The Knowledge and Skills Framework[10] aims to:

> Support the effective learning and development of individuals and teams – with all members of staff being supported to learn throughout

their careers and develop in a variety of ways, and being given the resources to do so.

This process provides new opportunities for developing careers in the NHS, with the focus on evidence of competence being of prime importance. Clinical supervision is one mechanism where the developmental needs of practitioners can be identified and acknowledged when achieved.

The HPC will require Allied Health Professionals (AHPs) to demonstrate their professional development through the proposed CPD standards[11] which require evidence of continued professional progression. Clinical supervision is advocated in current government policies as a useful tool for continuing professional development.[12]

Origins of clinical supervision

The origin of supervision within health and social care has been primarily from its use in psychological and mental health settings. The development of counselling has also shaped the outcome in terms of the models and approaches to supervision. Much of the research has been undertaken within nursing.[13] In the National Health Service the history of supervision is relatively recent. Professionals have been encouraged to integrate supervision into practice since the early 1990s. This has been driven by government initiatives such as *A First Class Service*.[4] There is a significant literature within nursing, describing the use and implementation of supervision, generally exhorting nurses to approach supervision positively. There is an assumption in much of the literature that supervision is good for developing clinical practice.[14] There is also some evidence that supervision can be seen as a coping strategy in order to manage stress in the work environment.[15]

Within occupational therapy there has been an expectation of undertaking supervision in practice since the 1970s. This was provided to students formally as part of their assessed placement experience and by 'good' managers to newly qualified staff. There was no formal training but the expectation that approaches learnt in mental health settings as part of pre-registration education would be effective in practice. This exposure to supervision as students and as practitioners has led occupational therapists to make assumptions about the knowledge and understanding of supervision in practice. The notion that the experience of educational supervision pre-graduation and skills used with clients equip occupational therapists with a framework of transferable skills to undertake clinical supervision in practice without further training needs challenging. Although occupational therapists have a history of using clinical supervision there remain questions about the quality of what takes place. It is, however, important to acknowledge that the conversation is taking place and is becoming more searching and challenging. There are other groups within the AHPs where this conversation is yet to take place.

Definitions of clinical supervision

The Department of Health[16] stated that clinical supervision is:

> A formal process of professional support and learning which enables the individual practitioners to develop knowledge and competence,

assume responsibility for their own practice and enhance consumer protection and safety of care in complex clinical situations.

Bond and Holland[14] describe supervision from a nursing perspective:

> Clinical supervision is regular, protected time for facilitated, in-depth reflection on clinical practice. Its aim is to enable the supervisee to achieve, sustain and creatively develop a high quality of practice through the means of focused support and development.

The Nursing and Midwifery Council (NMC)[17] supported the use of supervision:

> Clinical supervision is a practice focused professional relationship that enables you to reflect on your practice with the support of a skilled supervisor. Through reflection you can further develop your skills, knowledge and enhance your understanding of your own practice.

The Chartered Society of Physiotherapy (CSP) guidelines[18] stated that:

> Clinical supervision can be seen as a collaborative process between two or more practitioners of the same or different professions. This process should encourage the development of professional skills and enhanced quality of patient care through the implementation of an evidence-based approach to maintaining standards in practice. These standards are maintained through discussion around specific patient incidents or interventions using elements of reflection to inform the discussion.

Within occupational therapy, a North American perspective is that:

> Clinical supervision is defined as a specific aspect of staff development dealing with the clinical skills and competencies of each staff member. The structure for clinical supervision is typically one-to-one and/or small groups on a regular basis.[19]

The UK perspective, on the other hand, locates clinical supervision within service quality and governance, and professional development and lifelong learning in the *Professional Standards for Occupational Therapy Practice*.[20]

Perceptions of clinical supervision

Views of professional bodies

The College of Occupational Therapists (COT) has defined supervision for the pre-registration programmes, described as:

> Active work-based learning is enhanced and developed through reflection on, and critical evaluation of, practice, and by making links between theory and practice.[21]

The statement on lifelong learning[6] also stresses the importance of the continuing personal and professional development.

The CSP positively promotes the use of clinical supervision[22] within the context of CPD. These guidelines clearly delineate the process of development of clinical supervision for use by managers, clinical governance co-ordinators and CPD co-ordinators. The CSP guidelines encourage the use of supervision but there is limited recognition of the potential problems and difficulties within the process or relationships.

The Royal College of Speech and Language Therapists[23] locates clinical supervision within CPD and the British Dietetics Association[24] focuses on the reflective process informing the individual's CPD. It would appear that the use of clinical supervision is still in development in many areas of healthcare practice.

There appear to be significant differences in how AHP professional bodies promote and articulate the use of supervision in practice. This may be in relation to differing traditions of practice, or different levels of priority and emphasis given to clinical supervision as an approach to lifelong learning.

Evidence from the literature

Sweeney[25] identifies significant issues in how OTs manage clinical supervision which relate to role confusion, the uniprofessional and hierarchical nature of the structures that currently exist in the profession. The relationship is often uncomfortable and not effective at meeting the developmental needs of novice professionals, and the tensions in attempting to deliver this through a 'democratic' approach leave the supervisee struggling for direction and leadership. The recommendations from this research include training for supervisee and supervisor, exposure to models and theories of supervision, the adoption of suitable supervisory strategies, and, finally, supervision for the supervisor. The training and ongoing supervision of supervisors are also stressed by Butterworth et al.[13]

Sweeney[25] also suggests the use of mentoring to facilitate professional role modelling and peer support groups to provide the more informal needs of the therapist. A significant point is also made by Sweeney that given the amount of time that is allocated for clinical supervision within practice, there needs to be a greater evidence base to ensure the time is used productively, as opposed to going through the motions of a required ritual.

A more challenging view of clinical supervision is described by Gilbert[26] from a nursing perspective. He critiques the use of supervision and reflection as a tool for the surveillance of staff and of the control professional groups. This article suggests that we have failed to recognise how this control over health professionals impacts on the service that is provided to clients. He describes supervision and reflection as 'meticulous rituals of confessional' as a way of self-monitoring and disciplining professional practice. He suggests that professions are limited in their ability to challenge or shape their role in society because of these professionally imposed structures. He questions the value of these mechanisms and the concept of the autonomous practitioner in this context and believes that it is naïve to assume that clinical supervision is a good thing.

The unconscious psychological processes, such as transference and countertransference, involved in the supervisory relationship need to be acknowledged. An understanding of these concepts is important when exploring clinical supervision. Bond and Holland[14] briefly describe transference as:

> The supervisee's displacement of their own internal feelings onto the supervisor.

This could equally apply to the supervisor. Understanding these processes will support the development of a more insightful and considered approach to supervision. The significance of the supervisory relationship is exemplified by Butterworth et al.[13] as:

> The alliance between supervisor and supervisee is analogous to the therapeutic alliance, defined as the bond between nurse and patient which is necessary for the practice of high quality nursing.

An awareness of the levels of anxiety created by supervision is apparent from research in nursing, and there is evidence that resistance to clinical supervision aims to protect individuals from anxieties generated by the supervisory relationship.[14]

Butterworth et al.[13] also describe the 'glass head' syndrome, and this is a situation I have also encountered, where the supervisee thinks the experienced practitioner can read their mind. A fantasy about the omnipotence of the supervisor, but unhelpful when the aim is to facilitate clinical reasoning!

One of the main reasons for undertaking supervision is the performance management of staff, but this may not be expressed overtly. As Baptiste[27] states:

> Supervision however will remain within the arena of performance, ensuring the meeting of employment or professional expectations.

Not acknowledging the potential tension between accountability and personal development is one of the main areas of difficulty within clinical supervision.

Purpose of clinical supervision

Kadushin[28] describes the three main functions of supervision as educative, supportive and managerial. Supervision has three functions: formative, which is mainly educational; normative, which focuses on the policy, organisation and evaluation; and restorative, including debriefing with both positive and negative feedback on practice.

Hawkins and Shohet[29] have developed this further and describe supervision within four categories:

1 tutorial, which focuses on educational function but may include supportive and managerial elements
2 training supervision, where the function of supervision is normative or managerial
3 managerial supervision, which relates to hierarchical line management
4 consultancy supervision for experienced practitioners.

Butterworth et al.[13] argue that supervision provides a way of protecting nurses from burnout and work-related stress. However, it is suggested that:

> Attempts are being made to relate the impact of clinical supervision to patient outcome.

Butterworth et al.[13] reinforce the performance management aspect of supervision, rather than the more supportive and educative function.

An understanding of the processes involved in learning as adults is important to connect with the learning that can take place within supervision. This learning is defined by Knowles[36] as:

> The process of adults gaining knowledge and expertise.

Knowles focuses on the adult's control over the learning process and identified four phases in the adult learning process.

1 **Need:** Determine what learning is needed so as to achieve goals.
2 **Create:** Create a strategy and resources to achieve the learning goal(s).
3 **Implement:** Implement the learning strategy and use the learning resources.
4 **Evaluate:** Assess the attainment of the learning goal and the process of reaching it.

These phases can be compared to the processes implicit within successful clinical supervision.

It is useful to understand the stages in knowledge development as described by Dreyfuss.[31] The acquisition of knowledge through theory and experience helps us to explain to novice practitioners that there is a developmental process which they will need to explore. This may also help them to evaluate for themselves where they are in the process and provides a basis for a discussion.

- Novice uses established rules to function.
- The Advanced Beginner adapts learned rules to a context.
- The Competent Learner uses rules and context to formulate plans.
- The Proficient Learner uses intuition to make decisions.
- The Expert Learner uses practical wisdom in conjunction with intuition that is taken to a higher level.

Reflective practice

As already discussed, the role of reflective practice is often seen as crucial within clinical supervision. We are required to be reflective practitioners by our professional and statutory regulatory bodies. Therefore an understanding of our personal approach to reflective practice and the role of reflection is necessary when developing an appropriate approach to clinical supervision. Reflection within clinical supervision can provide an opportunity for progression and development in practitioners' understanding and practice.

The reflective process has been described by Kolb[32] as an experiential learning cycle, encompassing all stages of life, 'whereby knowledge is created through the transformation of experience'. Schon[33] made an important contribution to the understanding of reflection, developing the concepts of reflection in and on action, where practitioners attempt to make sense of unique practice experiences. There is a debate about these concepts but Schon recognised the centrality of practical experience as critical to the development of professional knowledge and understanding. He was primarily concerned about the gap between research-based knowledge and practice. In describing the reflective practitioner he identified the importance of practice-based knowledge which encouraged a significant shift in perspectives.

The reflective model that Boud and Knights[34] described includes the preparation, the experience and the reflective process. This places the reflective process in context of the experience, and stresses the importance of attending to the feelings generated in the situation. They describe learning as being located in the personal foundations of experience of the learner, 'those experiences that have shaped the person and helped to create the person he or she is now'.

An approach to reflection, incorporating and developing Schon's work, was designed for teacher and health visitor education by Fish *et al.* and identifies four strands within the reflective process.[35]

1 The factual strand: 'setting the scene, telling the story, pin-pointing critical events, identifying views about future practice'.
2 The retrospective strand: 'looking back over the entire events and processes of the practice as a whole and seeing patterns and possible new meanings in them'.
3 The substratum strand: 'uncovering and exploring critically the personal theory which underlies the piece of practice, and considering how it relates to and might be helped by formal theory'.
4 The connective strand: 'considering how present theory and practice might relate to future theory and practice, drawing on propositional knowledge'.

The substratum and the connective strands have been developed particularly to address the development of practice within clinical supervision.[36]

There are many ways to engage in reflective practice, for example, individually or in groups, using reflective journals or diary. The focus for this chapter has been to locate this in clinical supervision.

Who should carry out supervision?

Generally in healthcare supervision is undertaken within a line management arrangement, where junior staff are supervised by a member of staff more senior to them. The random nature of these relationships and the general absence of choice in the selection of supervisor reinforces the managerial, performance monitoring focus. The other important variable is that although a practitioner may be an excellent clinician, they may not have the necessary skills to supervise others appropriately. There needs to be a framework to structure and guide the process, not just to protect those involved but also to assist in the development of practice. Van Ooijen[37] states that newly qualified staff need to receive supervision from:

> Someone from the same professional background or theoretical orientation.

Concern about the inappropriateness of line managers undertaking the clinical supervisors role is supported by Bond and Holland[14] leading to:

> Restrictive practice rather than reflective and growthful practice.

This was amplified in the findings from Sweeney's research.[25]

However, for more experienced practitioners, supervision from a practitioner outside of one's own specialty can enhance professional development through the inclusion of different theoretical frameworks:

Experiencing supervision from people from different theoretical backgrounds can greatly facilitate such integration.[37]

Approaches to supervision

Given the variety of practice settings that exist in health and social care today the
aim is to create an approach which will be flexible but with clear boundaries, thus
setting a framework for practice progression. The selection of an appropriate
framework will depend on the demands of the setting and the perceptions of need
by the individuals involved. There are a variety of approaches which are briefly
outlined for you to consider.

Developmental approach

This approach to supervision in counselling is described by Hawkins and Shohet[29]
as four levels of supervisee development, focusing on education and development.

- **Level one:** Self-centred, as a novice who is dependent on their supervisor and
  requiring a structured framework for supervision which may also include an
  element of assessment.
- **Level two:** Client-centred, where the supervisee has gained a level of confidence and has moved on from the simply descriptive understanding of events.
  At this level the supervisee begins to struggle with their developing professional maturity, 'fluctuating between dependence and autonomy'.
- **Level three:** Process-centred, the supervisee is able to respond more appropriately to clients with a broader repertoire and a sound understanding of the
  client context.
- **Level four:** Process in context-centred, 'not about acquiring new knowledge,
  but allowing this to be deepened and integrated until it becomes wisdom'.

Using this developmental approach supports the progression of understanding
and knowledge, working from the level of understanding the supervisee has, and
integrates the experiential elements of practice into professional development.
Difficulties can be experienced by the supervisee when the level of expectation by
the supervisor is not accurately focused on the level of knowledge and experience
of the supervisee.[37]

The three steps method

Van Ooijen[37] has developed a practical and flexible framework which can be
applied in most settings. It outlines the 'what', the 'how' and the 'what now' of
supervision, which parallels the Donabedian[38] use of structure, process and
outcome.

- **Step 1:** The 'what' of the working alliance. Identifies the boundaries of the
  relationship between the supervisee and supervisor including an understanding of their feelings about each other, their professional role, their experience,
  and purpose and expectations of supervision.

- **Step 2:** The 'how' of a working agreement. Practicalities such as agreeing to work together, confidentiality and safety, accountability, resolving disputes, evaluation and timeframe.
- **Step 3:** The 'what now' of the working agreement. It is recommended that this step is used to design a written agreement having reflected on the previous two steps and based on feelings about the 'other' person, agreeing goals, the process of supervision, and what the commitment in the supervision is.

These three steps are then used to structure and review the implementation and progress of the supervisory relationship.

The double matrix or eight-eyed supervisor model

This model that Hawkins and Shohet[29] have developed is a process model of supervision from the counselling and psychotherapy tradition.
    The therapy session is reported and reflected upon in supervision.

1 Reflection on the content of the therapy session.
2 Exploration of the strategies and interventions used by the therapist.
3 Exploration of the therapy process and relationship.
4 Focus on the therapy process as it is reflected in the supervision process.
5 Focus on the supervisee's transference.
6 Focus on the here-and-now process as a mirror or parallel of the there-and-then process.
7 Focus on the supervisor's counter-transference.
8 Focus on the wider context.

The different elements within the framework are reflected upon in a structured manner to identify issues that need further exploration.

The growth and support model[13]

This model, from a nursing framework, focuses on the role of the supervisor in facilitating growth, 'both educationally and personally in the supervisee' and importantly to 'support their developing clinical autonomy'. The elements of this framework require the supervisor to have insight into: generosity, rewarding, openness, willingness to learn, thoughtful and thought-provoking, humanity, sensitivity, uncompromising, personal, practical, orientation, relationship and trust.

- **Confidentiality:** Clinical supervision should take place within a relationship where: 'Supervisors must establish an atmosphere of uncompromising confidentiality, trust and professionalism'.[13]
- **Supervision contracts:** This should provide a transparent and safe framework for the supervision to take place. Carrol, cited in Hawkins and Shohet,[29] describes four principles to be discussed:
    - practicalities
    - working alliance
    - presenting in supervision
    - evaluation.

The contract should be a clear written statement, discussed and agreed by the supervisee and supervisor, which is reviewed regularly.

Evaluation of supervision

Exploring how evaluation of clinical supervision should take place, van Ooijen[37] suggests some questions regarding the supervisee experience.

- How effective has the session been?
- What might have helped to make it more effective?
- What might need looking at further?
- What has not been reflected on?
- What is still not clear?

The same questions could also be asked from a supervisor's perspective, as a way of evaluating from the same framework. It is important to be mindful that there are anxieties about performance from the supervisee's and the supervisor's perspective. Hawkins and Shohet[29] suggest that evaluation should be a two-way process and that there are regular stocktaking times with feedback from both parties. The timing of evaluation will depend on the circumstances of the supervisory relationship, but will need to be discussed when the contract is first agreed. There have been some attempts to evaluate the use of clinical supervision in terms of staff satisfaction, but these have proved too complex to draw conclusions from.

What happens when supervision is not working?

Hawkins and Shohet[29] suggest exploring issues of concern within the supervisory relationship and to try to depersonalise this before seeking assistance from others. Experience shows the relationship can break down from either side and there need to be support mechanisms in place for both parties. How this is managed will depend on how mature the organisational culture is in the practice setting. Given the volume of change in practice this may be difficult to manage effectively.

Conclusion

The quest in clinical supervision has been to develop an effective, empowered and equitable approach for each of the participants in the supervisory relationship. As we move into a more in-depth appreciation of the complex nature of the supervisory relationship with its inherent tensions, the uncritical acceptance of supervision as a 'good thing' has ceased. The need to educate practitioners and managers in the giving and receiving of supervision is apparent. The gains from appropriate and effective supervision are manifold, for practitioners and service users alike.

The search for other ways of supporting development also need to be considered. Mentoring has been used in healthcare in an educational capacity for a range of practitioners. This approach could be used to broaden the support and development opportunities available. It is also potentially open to the same abusive power relationships as clinical supervision, but by including this in a transparent framework the danger of this will be reduced. The reasons for undertaking clinical supervision need to be clear to all involved, and the more transparent the process, the better. Other ways of supporting staff could include informal peer support groups.

Developing interprofessional approaches to the delivery and implementation of clinical supervision would open the process to scrutiny from differing perspectives and could potentially strengthen the process. Through the prism of my own experience, as a practitioner, manager and now educator, I pose the question 'are we getting it right?' and I suggest the answer is 'only in part'. The central concern relates to the quality of clinical supervision in practice, and to date there are no easy ways of assessing this from the practice or managerial perspective. The relationships formed through clinical supervision are subject to serendipity, with little focus on educating practitioners and managers to use this mechanism skilfully. The search is on for a way out of the 'matrix'.

References

1 *Learning from Bristol: the report of the public inquiry into children's heart surgery at the Bristol Royal Infirmary 1984-1995*. Command Paper: CM 5207. London: Stationery Office; 2001.
2 *The Royal Liverpool Children's Inquiry*. London: House of Commons; 2001.
3 Department of Health. *The New NHS: modern, dependable*. London: Department of Health; 1997.
4 Department of Health. *A First Class Service: quality in the new NHS*. London: Department of Health; 1998.
5 Department of Health. *Health Service Circular: Clinical Governance*. London: HMSO; 1999.
6 College of Occupational Therapists. *Position Statement on Lifelong Learning*. London: COT; 2002.
7 Department of Health. *NHS Plan*. London: HMSO; 2000.
8 Department of Health. *Meeting the Challenge: a strategy for the Allied Health Professions*. London: Stationery Office; 2000.
9 Department of Health. *Agenda for Change*. London: HMSO; 2004.
10 Department of Health. *The Knowledge and Skills Framework*. London: HMSO; 2000.
11 Health Professions Council. *Continuing Professional Development – consultation paper*. London: HPC; 2004.
12 Knutton S, Pover J. The importance of honesty in clinical supervision. *Nursing Management*. 2004; **10**: 9.
13 Butterworth T, Faugier J, Burnard P, editors. *Clinical Supervision and Mentorship in Nursing*. Cheltenham: Nelson Thornes; 1998.
14 Bond M and Holland M. *Skills of Clinical Supervision for Nurses*. Milton Keynes: Open University Press; 1998.
15 Craik C. Stress in occupational therapy: how to cope. *British Journal of Occupational Therapy*. 1988; **51**(2): 40–43.
16 Department of Health. *The Vision for the Future*. London: Department of Health; 1993.
17 Nursing and Midwifery Council. *Statement on Clinical Supervision*. London: NMC; 2001.
18 Chartered Society of Physiotherapy. *A Guide to Implementing Clinical Supervision For Qualified and Associate Members*. London: CSP; 2003.
19 Connecticut Certification Board; 1996. www.cot.org.uk (Accessed 27.1.2005).
20 College of Occupational Therapists. *Professional Standards for Occupational Therapy Practice*. London: COT; 2003.
21 College of Occupational Therapists. *Curriculum Framework for Pre-registration Education*. London: COT; 2004.
22 Chartered Society of Physiotherapy. *Mentoring*. CPD Information Paper No 35. London: Chartered Society of Physiotherapy; 2004.

23 Royal College of Speech and Language Therapy. 2005. www.rcslt.org.
24 British Dietetics Association.1998. www.bda.uk.com.
25 Sweeney G, Webley P, Treacher A. Supervision in occupational therapy. *British Journal of Occupational Therapy.* 2001; **64:** 7–9.
26 Gilbert T. Reflective practice and clinical supervision: meticulous rituals of confessional. *Journal of Advanced Nursing.* 2001; **36**(2): 199–205.
27 Baptiste S. *Mentoring and Supervision.* Canada: Canadian Association of Occupational Therapists; 2001.
28 Kadushin A. *Supervision in Social Work.* New York: Columbia University Press; 1976.
29 Hawkins P, Shohet R. *Supervision in the Helping Professions.* Milton Keynes: Open University Press; 2000.
30 Knowles M. *The Adult Learner.* Woburn MA: Butterworth-Heinemann; 1998.
31 Dreyfuss H, Dreyfuss S. *Mind Over Machine: the power of human intuition in the ear of the computer.* Oxford: Blackwell; 1986.
32 Kolb D. *Experiential Learning: experience as a source of learning and development.* New Jersey: Prentice Hall; 1984.
33 Schon D. *The Reflective Practitioner.* New York: Basic Books; 1987.
34 Boud D, Knights S. Course design for reflective learning. In: *Reflective Learning in Social Work.* Arena Publishing: Aldershot; 1993.
35 Fish D, Twinn S, Purr B. *Promoting Reflection: improving the supervision of practice in health visiting and initial teaching training.* Twickenham: West London Institute of Higher Education; 1991.
36 Twinn S, Johnson C. The supervision of health visiting practice. In Butterworth T, Faugier J, Burnard P, editors. *Clinical Supervision and Mentorship in Nursing.* Cheltenham: Nelson Thornes; 1998.
37 van Ooijen E. *Clinical Supervision Made Easy.* Edinburgh: Churchill Livingstone; 2004.
38 Donabedian A. Evaluating the quality of medical care. *Milbank Memorial Fund Quarterly.* 2005; **83**(4): 691.

Chapter 3

Teaching and learning for support staff: the critical issues

Sally Fowler-Davis, Christine Lynam and Anne Candelin

Why train support staff?

There is a strong probability that the characteristics of and skill mix within the local workforce have become an increasingly prominent issue for AHP managers, and that the recruitment of new types of support staff is key to meeting the recommendations laid out in the modernisation agenda. Crucial to the success of employing more staff who will work differently is the intention to educate and develop support staff to meet the diversity of needs within services. Workforce development planning now needs to take account of both registered and non-registered staff, who will all be contributing to services. They will need to be supported to fulfil an effective role within their service and to assess their own potential progression. It is possible that alongside Health Professions Council requirements for re-registration of qualified AHPs there will be a licensing procedure for support staff which will require them to produce evidence of their continuing development.

We hope to persuade the reader that the purpose and importance of support staff development have a wider strategic relevance than first it appears and that attention to this issue offers managers a model by which to configure a workforce to meet the changing needs of service and the personal advancement of individual staff. It is significant in moving forward the local modernisation agenda and potentially has a professional purpose in creating new roles and opportunities across the board.

The valuable role of support staff was stressed in *A Health Service of All the Talents: developing the NHS workforce*.[1] This emphasised the need to 'maximise the input and develop the skill of **all** . . . staff', as well as the need to encourage more flexible routes into professional training, particularly those which valued previous experience and knowledge.

Subsequently, *Meeting the Challenge: a strategy for the Allied Health Professions*[2] highlighted the need for support staff to have improved access to further training and development. This was reinforced in *Improving Working Lives for the Allied Health Professions and Health Care Scientists*[3] which stressed that:

> Career development should also be available to people who don't already hold professional qualifications.

During the period 2002–2005, the Department of Health (DH) developed and funded 12 pilot sites to investigate modernisation of the education and training for AHPs. As part of its bid, the College of York St John proposed the development of learning opportunities for staff at all levels, with particular reference to support staff. The successful bid promoted the idea of a 'stepping-stone' approach for those support workers with limited academic profiles. This was taken forward in the form of units of learning accredited through the Open College Network with over 89 support staff taking part and successfully achieving one or more credits. The experience of implementing the programme of learning opportunities has provided valuable insights into the needs of those embarking on study and is appropriate for the future development strategies for the management of learning for support staff working in a range of services.

One of the key aspects of the NHS modernisation agenda as outlined in *Modernising Health and Social Care*[4] was the goal of:

> Widening access to health professional programmes by encouraging mature entries and applicants from within the service.

This requires educational institutions to explore initiatives for widening access to programmes and supporting non-traditional entrants. The provision to transfer between programmes of study, and change direction without having to 'start from the beginning', was seen as advantageous. The experience of support staff has shown that approximately 10% of those who achieved credits on the learning opportunities programme have subsequently commenced studies on a foundation degree or an in-service undergraduate programme for occupational therapy students. This further illustrates the potential for development of staff when opportunities arise.

The NHS Plan[5] outlined the concept of Individual Learning Accounts for staff without a professional qualification and mentioned the new role of assistant practitioners for whom new programmes of education and training would be required.

Such a programme should also provide specifically tailored learning opportunities for that group of staff, in order to encourage engagement in learning, enhancement of knowledge and skills in the workplace and role development. This is consistent with the findings of the Audit Commission,[6] which stated:

> Managers and therapists need to maximise the use of skills by using assistants and helpers and by deploying qualified therapists more flexibly.

All the issues related to new roles and to role redesign are contained within the Career Framework,[7] which provides a flexible template for NHS organisations to redesign and adapt healthcare roles to achieve a modern workforce. It proposes basing job design on skills and competences required, rather than their need to fit solely with a particular profession. It also suggests eight career levels:

- Level 1: initial entry level jobs
- Level 2: support workers (healthcare assistants)
- Level 3: senior healthcare assistants
- Level 4: assistant practitioners/associate practitioners
- Level 5: practitioners
- Level 6: senior practitioners/specialist practitioners

- Level 7: consultant practitioners
- Level 8: more senior staff with the ultimate responsibility for clinical caseload decision making and full on-call accountability.

An illustration of this follows.

Box 3.1 Bolton Primary Care Trust

Bolton PCT was one year into a Greater Manchester SHA initiative to develop the role of assistant practitioner within the AHPs.

Trainee assistant practitioners spent two years developing experience of working with a number of different AHPs, nurses and social services staff, as appropriate to their new role. By illustration, in learning disability services they will have had placements covering speech and language therapy, physiotherapy, occupational therapy and nursing.

Assistant practitioners took on some of the responsibilities of practitioners, who in turn developed their roles by supporting other clinical staff such as junior doctors.

There was a 'fit' with the Knowledge and Skills Framework[8] and AHPs were encouraged to work in new and joined-up ways that will help to improve patient care. The fact that it was also a great motivator can only reinforce this message. The role of assistant practitioner, for example, provided a good stepping stone for those who eventually wanted to become qualified practitioners.[9]

The roles of assistant practitioner and advanced practitioner are both new roles and intended to address skills gaps by promoting new ways of working. This involves managers in role redesign: creating new roles, career progression and expanding the depth and breadth of roles, or moving tasks up or down a traditional unidisciplinary ladder.[10] In this process of redesign there is an argument to be made for the complementary development of education and training opportunities required to fulfil these roles and see them as offering the opportunities for individuals to progress. It is implicit in this argument that even those who wish to retain a current way of working will need development opportunities and, within the ever-changing skills demand, support staff will need encouragement and motivation to retain their competency. It is intended that the 'new type of worker' will pursue the organisation's goals and have a direct impact on service delivery whilst allowing professional practitioners to move practice forward through consultancy posts and extended-scope advanced practitioner posts.

Whilst the subject of this chapter is training and educational opportunities for support staff, of particular note here is recognition of the potential mobility and flexibility of the proposed assistant practitioner, a key role which is considered a crucial aspect for the delivery of future services. For individuals with valuable life experience, health and social care skills but no formal qualifications, educational opportunities arising from within the workplace offer a real possibility for the recognition of achievement. Such a reward is consistent with the belief that education is a life-enhancing experience. What is not on offer is the promise of vastly enhanced salaries.

The NHS is gradually realising the requirement of ongoing and embedded learning (for example e-learning, *see* Chapter 6) to meet the range of expectations both internal and external to the organisation. This is leading to a greater aspiration to integrate educational method in practice and to develop leaders who can make use of the 'knowledge culture' in the development of clinical practice and service delivery. Higher education is able to participate in a range of innovations relating to the provision of knowledge in terms of research implementation, staff/workforce development and the identification and leadership of change in the learning culture. *The NHS Plan*[5] was a deliberate and clear strategic document to unite the NHS under a corporate objective and mission and this was linked to the development of learning by all staff. *Agenda for Change*[11] denotes responsibility, status and pay for all employees alongside the specific responsibility (within each job and role) for the development of people. As such the NHS has the challenge of creating a 'learning organisation',[12] which is the ability and commitment to harness and extend collective learning in pursuit of strategic goals.

This idea and, some would argue, 'ideal' relies on the following principles: that education is intrinsically motivating and dignifying, is guided by individual choice and is an intentional activity to enhance knowledge. The process of learning in an organisation needs to become prominent but not dominant and requires supportive and consistent leadership, with leaders being prepared to engage with their own learning and to learn in their own practice.

Learning has an impact on staff, on services and on the individual who undertakes the educational opportunity. There is no doubt that education is a powerful change agent, especially for those who have had little or no access. If this can be harnessed by services for the benefit of patients, it is possible to consider learning as a strategy to enhance retention of staff and to recruit to all levels of service delivery by adopting a 'grow your own' policy to staffing.

It is also true that the demands placed on a service are often conflicting and pressurised and are likely to militate against learning opportunities for support staff. There are the competing priorities of service provision on a day-to-day basis, targets, waiting lists or time out for staff to develop their knowledge and skills. It is difficult to fulfil the needs of everyone concerned. However, work-based learning can go some way to benefiting both the service and the individual learner (*see* Chapter 5).

When talking to colleagues and service managers about learning for support staff it is common to hear a range of stories which come from one or two experiences about one or two individuals who have been supported in their development. The stories fall into two categories: first, a focus on the achievement of the person and their progression out of the service and second, the example of staff who, having experienced education, for example undergraduate programmes, have become reluctant to participate in the service in the same way as previously and are asking questions and challenging practice that previously went unchallenged. Both anecdotes tend to reinforce the idea that learning results in a loss to service delivery, giving rise to comments such as:

Now she's in the third year, she's always questioning everything.

What is rarely recounted are the experiences of support staff who have undertaken learning which has developed them either personally, professionally or both, resulting in an advancement of service delivery locally. A follow-up study on in-service graduates from an occupational therapy programme showed that after five years, 97% continued to work within the geographical locality from where they were recruited onto the programme (follow-up study of graduates from the in-service occupational therapy programme 1997–2002 – unpublished).

Opportunities for services through developing support staff

There has been a wide variety of opportunities for support staff. This has taken a number of formats, ranging from informal in-service training resulting in local certificates of achievement to more formalised awards such as National Vocational Qualifications (NVQ). Competency-based training is based on job analysis and associated skills analysis. A job becomes a list of duties and tasks and the skills needed to perform the task can be described in specific detail. The ability to demonstrate those tasks and skills is viewed as a measure of competency and has been formalised within the structure of NVQs. This award has been questioned for being a performance, rather than a knowledge-based qualification. As such, there is no real aspect of development; it does not necessarily equate with new or improved performance, but is simply a validation of existing performance. This can result in motivational issues for participants, and questions about its purpose and validity.

For AHP support staff the qualification has proved unpopular and the rewards and relevance have been questioned. Currently, there are insufficient assessors and the requirements are overly time-consuming for both the learner and the assessor.

By contrast, knowledge-based training is called education or learning. It assumes that from knowledge comes the ability to think critically about how to undertake an activity, however simple or complex. Tasks are learned and practised and as new knowledge is applied, the person is able to perform the task more skilfully and is able to adapt to the specific demands of the environment. Such adaptation of performance is based on knowledge and the ability to appraise a range of information related to the activity and the environment in which it takes place.

The assessment of competence in performance seems, therefore, to require a number of key components: the testing of performance in at least one context, questioning about the underpinning principles of action and additional demonstration of tasks in a variety of contexts where they appear in the working role.

The key thing about the recognition of achievement is that, above all else, all qualifications need to have currency. They are valuable only when they can be transferred between organisations and sectors and have geographical portability. This obviously reduces the value of in-service training. The key to the provision of learning opportunities is the identification of learning needs, the structure for development and the commitment to seek out the strategies to implement learning, either formal or informal. This may be achieved in house or collaboratively with partners in education settings.

In suggesting that specific and accredited learning opportunities are made available for support staff, there is no intention to diminish the value of informal learning, which is the most commonly cited experience of development in support staff.[13] Workshops, study days, visits or other in-house learning opportunities and other informal learning can serve as a trigger to motivate the learner, validate practice and develop competence. Whether a service offers opportunities for informal or formal learning, there is a considerable degree of management required. One way forward can be the implementation of work-based learning strategies. Work-based learning involves exploring issues and problem solving with direct relevance to the participants' own workplace context. Any discussion on strategies and structures for the delivery of learning opportunities must be viewed in the context of award and qualification. In this respect, work-based learning is no exception. Awards mean different things to different types of workers. This is particularly true of support staff who have no specific work-related qualification and therefore no registration to a professional body or group.

Level of competence, frameworks for learning

Skills for Health was established in April 2002 but officially licensed on 1 June 2005, with support from the four UK health departments. Its role is to be a focus for development of skills across the UK in the NHS, the independent sector and charities who provide health or social care.

Skills for Health works closely with other sector skills councils (SSCs) across the government's Skills for Business network and aim to:

> Train a workforce in such a way that patients can gain quick access to people who have the right skills to suit their needs; staff have the opportunity to fulfil their potential and skills and competencies developed in one setting are recognised and transferable right across the UK.[14]

The work of Skills for Health is central to the strategic development of the health sector workforce. The content and breadth of the Skills for Health programme cover linkages with all major workforce development initiatives. They are to be responsible for the Department of Health educational quality assurance programme. Also, the Care Group Focus workforce teams who support the workforce development required to deliver the National Service Frameworks, is part of their work programme.

Its main role is to create and disseminate UK-wide competency frameworks which will underpin local training initiatives. The competency frameworks are based on an agreement between employers and training providers as to what skills and therefore learning are required to undertake a particular job. Part of Skills for Health's work is to establish sets of National Occupational Standards for staff in all areas of the health service. These describe what an individual is required to achieve. They can also help managers anticipate future recruitment and training needs and improve service delivery by having better trained staff.

> In theory, training in the NHS should operate like an Open University degree, where you build credits for every module you take and can move across from one professional strand to another.[14]

This is perceived as the way in which 'building blocks' of learning can be used in different areas of service and within different organisations based on recognised competencies. Skills for Health is focused on matching all levels of employment with competency-based training, which it believes proves the level of skill in the workforce, required to deliver health and social care services. This is operated through the development and dissemination of National Occupational Standards.

Whilst NVQ awards are clearly the dominant option at level 2 and 3 of the career framework, there has been a continuing discussion regarding the educational requirement at level 4 Assistant Practitioner and this has been linked to a newer award, namely the foundation degree. This is an intermediate academic award, which can be tailored to meet the needs of health and social care staff. It is achieved when participants have gained at least 240 higher education credits and is a nationally recognised vocationally oriented award in its own right, integrating both academic and work-based learning through close collaboration with employers and programme providers. Work-based learning can be cost-effective and makes good use of time and opportunity to link specifically into service delivery and is an integral part of foundation degrees, which are structured over two years full time or four years part time. During the first year they aim to provide the basic, generic requirements for those working in health and social care, for example communication, applied sciences, patient and carer focus. The second year is an opportunity to provide curriculum which is tailored to either a care group (for example, diabetes) or to a professional group (for example, radiography assistant practitioners). The planning of programmes has both regional and national dimensions and SHAs are continuing to make the decisions about commissioning the range of education provision to meet local workforce redesign based on collaboration with local employers.

Formal educational pathways require a previously underdeveloped partnership between higher education and further education providers and health employers but requires succession planning, fills skill gaps in service delivery and impacts on the quality of service provision. This has been demonstrated through in-service undergraduate programmes where graduates have returned to their services and fulfilled roles in both developing services and those that are traditionally short-staffed. Where a service is known to promote learning opportunities this can encourage recruitment and retention of staff.

Engaging support staff in learning

Support staff are a diverse learning group. On a practical level the scope of work role and responsibility can vary hugely. This in itself can be a source of tension in the learning environment due to inequalities in levels of responsibility, supervision and remuneration. Previous learning experience can range from higher qualifications to no formal learning since leaving school.

Aspirations include the motivation to learn for pleasure and interest, an escape from the workplace or to support ambition to access higher education. In the worst case scenario, learners can feel they have been 'made to learn'. This diversity manifests itself in attitudes such as excitement, resistance, anger, fear, overestimating or underestimating potential. Such attitudes must be carefully managed if learning is to be purposeful. As Minton[15] described this crucially involves engaging:

> . . . the student in the learning process . . . through taking an active role.

Instrumental to the achievement of such engagement is the need to support individuals through their fears and anxieties, explain the purpose of learning, nurture enthusiasm and most importantly make the explicit links between knowledge-based learning, the individual work role and crucially the individual themselves.

Embarking on study can provoke a range of reactions from individuals. It should not be forgotten that for some learners their only previous experience of learning may have occurred at school with a pedagogical approach. The transition to andragogy and the concept of the independent learner can take time and careful management. Without this the learner can become discouraged and overwhelmed. To make that transition, learners should be encouraged to develop robust study skills.[16]

Achievement and recognition of learning by way of credits and sometimes certificates/diplomas/degrees are most importantly a reward for the individual, but also a public recognition of achievement. For some it will be the first opportunity to demonstrate ability to achieve set standards. For others it will be the stepping stone to reach future goals. A service which has supported a learner through the process can also be assured of recognition and development through having staff members who are up-to-date and motivated.

Any learning opportunities programme should emphasise the ongoing development of knowledge of therapy practice and skills and the underpinning scope of the role of support staff. It is important that it is managed to ensure purpose and relevance to the person and their role, enabling progression of skills and knowledge. For example, it is normal practice to engage support staff in discussion and sharing of information, explore options for action/treatment/work-related activities, and to encourage reflection and resolution of problems. These everyday activities create a learning environment within the workplace and add value to the input of staff. Through these informal arrangements it can become evident that there are specific learning needs and therefore the process of shaping staff development begins. The process of identifying a structure to support this learning is the more complex decision because of the range of considerations which the manager and staff need to take into account.

Unlike professional practitioners, competency for support staff is not the first level toward achieving mastery through expertise. However well a support staff member performs, he/she cannot progress beyond being competent. This is because in relation to unqualified status, competency is a judgement of skills, not knowledge in practice. It refers to the individual's skill in supporting the role of professional staff and in undertaking direct service delivery. The Knowledge and Skills Framework[17] attempts to define skills, competencies and performance levels related to all jobs within the NHS. As such it aims to represent these features across a spectrum and suggests a measurable standard of skills. Competence in relation to support staff has commonly referred to the basic ability required to perform a task under supervision.

Establishing learning needs and opportunities

It is necessary to determine the levels of competence required to undertake specific tasks and roles and to distinguish this from ongoing learning opportunities, which encourage the learner to achieve greater knowledge and skills to broaden the scope of their practice. The modernisation pilot project (2002–05) (School of Professional Health Studies Project report – 2005 Modernising Pre-registration Education for the Allied Health Professions, Physiotherapy and Occupational Therapy (unpublished)) identified two sets of competencies: core competencies and those competencies related to specific care groups. As can be seen, this enabled identification of competencies shared by occupational therapy and physiotherapy professions and those specific to each profession (*see* Table 3.1).

As a starting point this workshop exercise demonstrated a potential structure for the development of a learning programme which had the potential to be appropriate for more than one profession. It has now been superseded by the Knowledge and Skills Framework[17] but was consistent with the concept of a continuum of learning from informal provision through to formal programmes with awards and professional status.

Formal learning by way of courses, modules or programmes is normally facilitated through educational institutions. Further options for learning can be investigated or initiated either by individual staff or by managers of services on their behalf. The most important first step is to identify what is required and how it will be supported through funding, time available and resource. It has to be recognised that the learner and the service will incur additional pressures when embarking on a programme of study and questions should be asked before commitment is finalised.

Considerations for managers of AHP services

The considerations outlined below are consistent with leading a learning community where a facilitator method is required to achieve the goals of learning participation and achievement. This is not an opportunity for 'command and control' but rather the encouragement of participation and active learning and sharing of knowledge at every level. The commitment to provide learning for support staff personnel needs to be underpinned by some of the principles common to learning organisations. This may help counteract some of the difficulties encountered in management and make learning a strategic driver to development and change. Staff need to feel encouraged to learn and to share learning and learn as a team and the manager might consider 'knowledge-in-practice' as the cement holding the organisation together. Attitudes to learning can be coloured by previous experience like school, and this may be a considerable barrier to engaging staff in new learning

In *Developing Professional Knowledge and Competence* Eraut[18] suggests that any framework for promoting learning needs to include a number of factors: a combination of learning settings – home, library, college, work, time for study, time for consultation and time for reflection, and people who are prepared to coach/teach/support the learner. Whilst these factors are common in the educational environment, to implement them successfully in the workplace, a full range of support mechanisms is required. Many academic providers will facilitate additional training in mentoring and supporting staff in the workplace which then has transferability to a range of work-related learning contexts. In addition, organisations can also support placement opportunities for those participants seeking careers in health and social care.

Table 3.1 Competencies for support staff

Occupational therapy	Physiotherapy
To provide a variety of interventions under supervision from professional staff.	To provide a variety of interventions under supervision from professional staff.
To manage a caseload delegated by professional staff.	To manage a caseload delegated by professional staff.
Undertaking assessments/screening with supervision and guidance from professional staff.	Undertaking assessments/screening with supervision and guidance from professional staff.
Monitoring, supervising and following up clients and patients.	Monitoring, supervising and following up clients and patients.
Responsible for routine organisation, clerical, administrative and domestic tasks relating to the running of the service.	Responsible for routine organisation, clerical, administrative and domestic tasks relating to the running of the service, e.g. referral, information gathering and circulation, departmental tidiness and cleanliness.
Supporting the work of the qualified staff.	Support the work of the qualified staff.
Working autonomously when required.	Act as patient advocate.
	Work autonomously when required.

Core competencies	Core competencies
Understand the ethics, theories, values and culture of the profession.	Understand the requirements and priorities of the organisation: policies, procedures and protocols.
Understand the requirements and priorities of the organisation: policies, procedures and protocols.	Implement the statutory requirements of Health and Safety training at all times.
Implement the statutory requirements of Health and Safety training at all times.	Develop a range of communication skills required in a variety of situations.
Develop a range of communication skills required in a variety of situations.	Understand the qualities of effective and appropriate communication styles.
Understand the qualities of effective and appropriate communication styles.	Know the criteria for service provision.
Know the criteria for service provision.	Understand and support the role of professional staff.
Understand and support the role of professional staff.	Understand basic anatomy, physiology and psychology applied to human functioning and patient conditions.
Understand basic anatomy, physiology and psychology applied to human functioning and client conditions.	Use a range of physiotherapy treatment media and equipment relevant to patient needs and as directed by professional staff.
Understand the criteria for planning and implementing a variety of creative, practical and technical media relevant to client needs and service provision.	

Table 3.1 *cont.*

Core competencies	*Core competencies*
Maintain and respect confidentiality at all times.	Know and use a range of resources.
Understand the principles of time management, prioritisation and caseload management.	Understand the principles of confidentiality and consent and maintain these principles at all times.
Know and use a range of resources.	Know limitation of knowledge, skill and role and when to seek advice.
Skills	**Skills**
Use numeracy and literacy skills.	Use numeracy and literacy skills.
Use problem-solving and decision-making skills.	Use problem-solving and decision-making skills.
Demonstrate, present and teach appropriately and effectively.	Demonstrate, present and teach appropriately and effectively.
Plan, develop, lead and adapt treatment sessions with individuals and groups.	Plan, develop, lead and adapt treatment sessions with individuals and groups.
Use observation skills and make appropriate judgements.	Use observation skills and make appropriate judgements.
Use skills of assessment as required, e.g. risk.	Use skills of assessment as required, e.g. risk.
Use communication and interpersonal skills effectively.	Use communication and interpersonal skills effectively.
Choose and implement a range of media using activity analysis and application principles.	Demonstrate organisational, time management and administrative skills.
Demonstrate organisational, time management and administrative skills.	Contribute appropriately to supervision and support.
Contribute appropriately to supervision and support.	**Other**
	Common sense.
	Sense of humour.
	Able to cope with patients' personality.
	Trustworthy.
	Professional.
	Knowing boundaries
	Legal issues.

Providing educational opportunities assumes that other strategic objectives for staffing have been considered. Developing a person assumes that the organisation has ambition for them to question and challenge operational assumptions and the way that they undertake routine tasks. It is likely that a new pattern to practice will emerge and they must be allowed to operate in new ways. For staff to be empowered by education and then told to maintain routine, unquestioning bureaucratic or mechanical tasks is not only wasteful of everyone's effort but profoundly demoralising of the potential for change in the organisation.

Managing a service must include the development of senior staff to support and innovate alongside support staff. This is consistent with the Knowledge and Skills Framework which requires higher level staff to contribute to the development of others. In doing so there will be benefits to individuals either as recipients of or as developers of learning and to the service as a whole; the development of team approaches is more consistent with learning environments than hierarchies. The tendency to make wide distinction between qualified and professional, and unqualified and by reference 'unprofessional' is strong and needs to be curbed.

> In our department it is normal for qualified staff to sit together in coffee breaks and the support staff to do the same. I am not sure now as to which group I belong. I feel that I am not a support worker but I'm not a qualified therapist either so I don't belong in either group.
>
> Comment from a student

Learning will almost inevitably create resistance and fear that old and trusted ways will be lost. Helping each individual to absorb and understand the mission of the service and the organisation is the first challenge and underpins the learning process – so-called network intelligence.

For some services a programme of enabling successive staff to enter programmes of study has facilitated future planning and development of the service, with the assurance of available staff with the appropriate skills to fill the positions. Collaborations between services, higher education institutions (HEI) and further education organisations are being established with the shared ambition of meeting the evolving needs of the modernised service. The consideration of what roles support staff might take up as a result of their education is critical to the wider development of the service.

Skill mix, within professional services or care groups, can be enhanced by increasing the role diversity of a team. There is a need to manage the new tension which comes from people being empowered and asking questions. Where support staff are in limited and technical roles, they may become frustrated with their positions and duties if educated to perform from a point of increased knowledge. This is a phenomenon which is frequently experienced by support staff studying on part-time undergraduate programmes where there is a conflict between the expectations placed on them as a student, particularly at the later levels of the programme, and the requirements of their ongoing work role.

For a manager attempting to support a learning culture within the workplace there may be many competing pressures and these need to be considered at an early stage in the process. It is our experience that support which is withdrawn subsequent to a member of staff applying for a course devalues both them and the place of learning within their organisation.

Releasing staff for dedicated learning time places demands on the service, while completing a programme of learning and its intended outcomes places demands on the individual. It is vital that there are realistic expectations from both the service and the individual as to what can be achieved and the time and effort required to do so within the context of work pressures.

> Now that I'm over half way through the course I can't give up, because I know too much to go back to being 'just a helper'. So I have no choice but to go on and that is sometimes an enormous pressure.
>
> Comment from a student

Possible solutions

Funding and finance

Of critical importance is the need to fund the delivery of learning, work-based learning is by no means resource free. SHA's should specifically be able to understand learner need in the health workforce. They are responsible for the commissioning and performance management of health education for undergraduate training and postgraduate CPD. They are also the body who allocates the Individual Learning Account (ILA), which at the time of writing is £150 per person per year and accessible by any health practitioner working inside or outside the National Health Service. These grants are paid directly to trusts on the basis of the workforce but AHP services have often been unaware of this resource, which is in addition to their training budget. Specific detail about the ILA is available from the SHA office and may be slightly different in each area about how the funds are allocated. Funding sources may also be suggested by the local or regional HEI and bids to the European Social Fund or alternative government departments may also be possible, jointly with the educational organisation.

Learning and assessment

We have found that 30-hour blocks of learning are manageable amounts of time for both the individual learner and for services. In this scenario, the 30-hour blocks can be split between dedicated 'teaching' time and individual learner activities.

However, this is not prescriptive in that shorter periods can be used, for example study days to promote specific learning such as pain management. Study days held locally can also provide opportunities for qualified staff to manage and deliver the learning thus fulfilling CPD as well as developing support staff and lowering costs. Should credits be required, the normal tariff is 10 hours = 1 credit.

Formal learning which attracts awards requires the evidence of achievement of the learning. This is normally demonstrated through the completion of assessment related to the learning. Assessment methods used with support staff learning are more appropriate if they are based on the workplace to enable the learner to integrate their learning within their post as well as having access to support from peers and managers. Most importantly, assessment must:

- be achievable within the resources available to the individual and service
- use a variety of methods, e.g. projects, case studies, evaluations, presentations, diaries, resource files, work-based examples

- bridge academic requirements and practice
- be easily updated and responsive to changing work demands and environments, for example consistent with the 'roll-out' of the modernisation agenda.

Most of all assessments must be clearly and explicitly relevant to the organisation and the individual, otherwise they will be viewed negatively as a 'hoop-jumping' exercise.

Accessibility of learning

When considering AHP support staff, learning can only be effective when it is accessible to the group for which it is intended. This involves developing learning opportunities that are:

- **At the appropriate learning level:** Experience of the modernisation project has indicated the need to consider the entry levels to learning to facilitate achievement and enhance motivation. This requires consideration of strategies to prepare the learner, e.g. introduction to study skills, as well as analysis of the amount and complexity of the learning to be achieved. To aim too high is anxiety provoking and demotivating, whereas to aim too low can appear patronising and lacking in justification. The importance of achieving the correct balance and preparing adequately cannot be overemphasised.
- **Applicable to a variety of work settings/differing roles:** The need to provide specific knowledge and programmes that can be relevant to staff within specific service areas/care groups lends itself most readily to content that is primarily knowledge based. The development of programme content must take into account a variety of key considerations: for example, the Knowledge and Skills Framework, and the diversity of support worker roles and responsibilities. There is a need to place emphasis on knowledge-based content which can be transferred and applied in a variety of settings.
- **Local venues:** The location of learning is significant on a number of levels. The choice of venue can impact negatively or positively on the learning process. Consistency of venue can be helpful in promoting a sense of security in learning which may help overcome some of the attitudinal barriers to learning. From our own experience, learners greatly value and benefit from learning outside of their immediate work environment. However, the venue's suitability must be matched with accessibility to learners. Prohibitive travel times and travel costs can quickly result in disengagement of the learner.
- **National accreditation and links with HEIs:** The role of higher or further education in the development of a sustainable support staff programme of learning and development would seem to be critical. It offers the opportunity for a service to access quality experience in assessment and quality monitoring which would be difficult to provide from the health and social care setting. Collaboration between HEI/further education and health/social care would utilise different methods. This may be difficult for a service manager who wishes to make links with a specific institution. However, as a common interest in support staff development is fuelled by modernisation and workforce development then it is likely to become easier to make the right contacts and progress a learning ambition.
- **Support for learners:** Many staff require preparation for learning and this

requires specialist support. A combination/synthesis of delivery approaches is generally required in order to meet a range of learning styles and requirements. Adult learners seem to appreciate the input of peers and peer supports[19] irrespective of level of study and this needs to be blended with independent study to achieve a creative approach to learning.

Comments from learners include:

> It was really interesting to meet people from other services and see the differences and similarities in our roles. This really added to the value of the learning and gave new insights.

> I feel that the module has validated what I do and this has built my confidence and made me want to learn more.

Box 3.2 Questions that managers should ask about learning development

Consideration of pressures such as:

1 Staffing levels to support study time and maintain service commitments. What will be the effect on service provision of releasing the staff member to undertake the study?
2 Funding. The costs of fees, textbooks, internet access, travel, possible accommodation can become high over a period of time. It is essential that the person and the manager have a realistic view of costs involved and decide at the outset who will be responsible for covering the cost of each element.
3 How will the outcomes of increased knowledge and skills be utilised within the service and what will (a) the service expect of the person and (b) the person expect of the service on successful completion of the learning?
4 Fairness in provision of learning opportunities.
5 What are the attendance and study requirements?
6 Would it be more manageable to facilitate local learning for staff groups rather than individuals in collaboration with education providers? If so, how many staff would be involved and how could this be designed to meet local needs?

Questions that learners should ask about learning development:

- How long is the programme/module/course?
- How is the proposed learning relevant to (a) my role and (b) the service?
- Will I be expected to cover any of the costs?
- How much study will be required, especially out of work time?
- Will this be manageable?
- What are the awards and how will I be able to use them in the future?
- Does the study fit in with my ambitions and aspirations?
- Will this change my relationships with my colleagues?
- What support will I get?

Conclusion

Lifelong learning, which is the fundamental driver to all that has been said in this chapter and which is a central concept of government policy for health improvement and workforce redesign. We endorse education as a 'right' for the individual and a primary force for change and development. If the power of education is to be harnessed by organisations, service or department then the management of this process and the link to both the organisational and individual goals must be overt and tangible. The role of an organisation is to respond to the external environment, using the human and non-human resources available. The NHS is both transforming itself and also having to understand the demands of a client group which are complex and sometimes conflicting and often politically driven. Learning within the organisation is critical to both individual public sector employees and also to the quality of service, if not the very survival of a publicly funded organisation.

In this respect we are strongly suggesting that in committing to a range of development opportunities for support staff, a manager is committing to other strategic developments of the service. A strategic goal for a service is likely to link with the development of staff at every level. Whilst this may be obvious, given that staffing is a major resource consideration for many managers, some have continued to see support staff development in the context of the individual and not a support for the business plan. This is all the more true when the learning needs of a group of support staff can be identified against a specific service development or an area of work where efficiencies can be demonstrated as a result.

Work-based learning has not been fully explored in this chapter and there are many texts which would support the manager in understanding the key differences between traditional theory-based education and other forms (*see* Chapters 5 and 6). Work-based learning is arguably a new challenge for HEIs and many professional health educators are now developing courses and programmes to link learning more closely with the workplace.

Critical to the development of support staff learning opportunities is the achievement of a synergy between the knowledge base and application in the workplace. Study skills can widen the horizons of an individual and demonstrate how knowledge and study do offer the euphemistically termed ladder of learning, taking the individual onto further study in recognised professions or in foundation subjects. In short, work-based learning appears to be effective when it adopts traditional modes of delivery – classroom/peer group/teachers and people.

SHAs are influenced by good practice initiatives which demonstrate modernisation and a clear needs analysis from service. This will be all the more powerful if the resource is local and demonstrates a link with the modernisation agenda for developing AHP services.

References

1 Department of Health. *A Health Service of All the Talents: developing the NHS workforce*. London: Stationery Office; 2001.
2 Department of Health. *Meeting the Challenge: a strategy for the Allied Health Professions*. London: Stationery Office; 2000.

3 Department of Health. *Improving Working Lives for the Allied Health Professions and Healthcare Scientists*. London: Stationery Office; 2002.

4 Department of Health. *Modernising Health and Social Care*. London: Stationery Office; 1999.

5 Department of Health. *The NHS Plan*. London: Stationery Office; 2000.

6 Audit Commission. *Hidden Talents: education, training and development for healthcare staff in NHS Trusts*. London: Audit Commission; 2000.

7 Department of Health. *Working Together, Learning Together: a framework for lifelong learning in the NHS*. London: Department of Health; 2001.

8 Department of Health. *NHS Knowledge and Skills Framework and the Development Review Process*. London: Department of Health; 2003.

9 www.dh.gov.uk/PublicationsAndStatistics/Bulletins/AlliedHealthProfessionalsBulletin (accessed 9 August 2005).

10 www.wise.nhs.uk/cmsWISE/Workforce+Themes/Using_Task_Skills_Effectively/roleredesign/Introduction/Introduction.htm (accessed 9 August 2005).

11 Department of Health. *Agenda for Change: modernising the NHS pay system*. London: Stationery Office; 1999.

12 Argyris C. *Knowledge in Action*. San Francisco: Jossey-Bass; 1993.

13 Fowler Davis S, Northrop J. *Developing Support Staff in the NHS*. Unpublished report for LSC Yorkshire NEYNL WDC; 2005.

14 Rogers J. Skills for Health. *HSJ Supplement*. 2005. **2 June**.

15 Minton D. *Teaching Skills in Further and Adult Education*. 2nd ed. London: Thompson Learning; 2005.

16 Lynam C. Teaching skills for health professionals. *Therapy Weekly*. 2005. **10 Nov**.

17 Department of Health. *NHS Knowledge and Skills Framework and the Development Review Process*. London: Stationery Office; 2004.

18 Eraut M. *Developing Professional Knowledge and Competence*. London: RoutledgeFalmer; 1994.

19 Chartered Society of Physiotherapy and College of Occupational Therapy. *A National Framework for Support Worker Education and Development*. London: CSP/COT; 2005.

Chapter 4

Management of student placements

Jane Morris and Ann Moore

Introduction

The main focus of this chapter is an overview of some of the current issues that have impacted on the education of students in the practice setting, highlighting recent and ongoing strategies that have been employed to manage placement education. The issues are initially explored at a macro level, enabling factors that impact on placement education nationally to be discussed together with recent and ongoing initiatives that have been employed to manage student placements. The final section focuses on the management and organisation of placements at a micro or local level, enabling practice education within trusts and the organisation of individual placements to be explored.

A range of placement models are identified and strategies for supporting educators in the practice setting are discussed. In addition, the ways in which the quality of placement learning is maintained are explored.

It has long been acknowledged that the education of students in the practice setting forms an essential part of all health professional courses, with experienced, health professionals being well placed to educate students within the practice learning environment. It is a mandatory requirement that all pre-registration health professional students are required to successfully complete a minimum of 1000 hours of supervised and assessed learning in the practice setting. Pre-registration students must therefore experience a range of different practice that requires them to integrate knowledge, skills and attitudes and to practise with a range of different people who have different needs.[1]

> Practice based learning forms an indispensable and integral part of the learning process. Learning gained in practice settings is vital to students' educational and professional development.[2]

The practice element of health professional pre-registration is facilitated and assessed by senior practitioners who fulfil their role as educators in the practice setting. This role is seen to be a crucial one, supporting the professional development of future generations of competent practitioners.

It is therefore essential that practice educators are supported by their colleagues in higher education and their managers in fulfilling this key role.[3]

Recent challenges to the provision of practice education

In recent years education providers have been required to increase student numbers in order to meet NHS workforce targets. In *The NHS Plan*[4] the government set out a plan to commission a substantial increase in pre-registration student numbers across health professional groups in an effort to meet workforce targets during the next decade. The planned increase from 15 600 physiotherapists in 2000 to 24 800 in 2009 equates to an increase of 59%, with similar figures being suggested for other health professionals groups. As a result of this sudden and considerable increase in pre-registration student numbers, both education providers and placement providers have faced significant challenges as they attempt to ensure that learners in the practice setting have access to sufficient numbers of placements that will enable them to gain the professional experience necessary to make them fit for practice, fit for purpose and fit for award.[5]

Although clinical placements have long been in short supply, the sudden recent surge in student numbers has made it increasingly more and more difficult to find adequate numbers of placements that enable pre-registration students to gain appropriate experience in the practice setting.[6,7]

Opportunities for exploring new models of placement education

In order to address the aforementioned challenges to placement provision, a number of higher education institutions in collaboration with education consortia and placement providers have explored different ways of addressing placement shortages. In recent years this has resulted in a number of collaborative projects being commissioned to explore and evaluate a range of different models of practice education.[5,7-9] This opportunity for university-based educators and placement providers to reflect on more traditional approaches to practice education and to explore different models has led to innovative ways of addressing practice learning being explored and tested. These have included the collaborative placement model, the role-emerging model,[8] the split placement model and the team model.[10,11]

Traditionally most undergraduate health professional pre-registration learners have experienced the 1:1 model of practice education, where one student is supervised by a senior health professional adopting the role of practice educator, who has responsibility for facilitating and assessing student learning in the practice setting. It has been widely acknowledged that the 1:1 model cannot continue to support the increasing demand for placements.[7,12] A study by Huddleston[8] questioned the wisdom of continued deliverance of a 1:1 model of practice education which may make students more reliant on their educators and lead to unrealistic expectations regarding the amount of support they will receive as newly qualified practitioners.

Collaborative placement models

In recent years a number of projects have evaluated the collaborative model placement supervision where two or more students are placed with one practice educator.[5,7,9,13]

A number of educational benefits for both learners and educators have emanated from the collaborative model of placement learning that promotes peer-assisted learning. These benefits have included the development of team skills and professional socialisation,[6] promotion of deep learning approaches[14] and the development of clinical reasoning skills.[15] Although the collaborative placement model, with its emphasis on peer-assisted learning, has long been accepted as the preferred method of delivering practice education in Australia, North America and Canada until recently the 1:1 placement model has remained the favoured method of placement delivery in the UK despite little evidence being around to support its continued use.

In recent studies undertaken in the UK both student and educator perceptions of the 2:1 model of placement learning were generally positive.[7]

Students have found the support from their peers invaluable as the following quotations from pre-registration students indicate:

> It's nice to be with someone who's in the same boat . . . or at the same level.

> It helps to bounce ideas back from each other so when you treat your patient, you know you haven't just got a couple of ideas, you've got more and you feel confident and, yeah, I think it really does help.

Students valued having a peer on placement with them and felt that the presence of another learner helped them to explore different approaches of patient management and enabled them to feel more confident in the practice environment. Students also found that by observing each other with patients and giving each other feedback the learning experience was enriched.

> I think we're quite good at feedback. If I come out of a situation and if I've been observed I feel quite happy asking X what they thought of it.

Educators also reported a number of benefits from having more than one student on placement in the same practice setting. For example, in the 2:1 model educators found their ability to demonstrate and practise treatment techniques was facilitated by having a second student on placement, as they had an additional person to use as a model. They also felt that learning and teaching sessions were more rewarding, as more discussion was generated and students tended to ask more questions that made them think about their practice and their own clinical reasoning.

> I know some people may say how can you cope with having two students . . . I quite enjoy it because it makes me think about what I'm doing . . . They tend to have more confidence to question you while you're doing things, which is no bad thing from my point of view. Keeps you on your toes. Makes you think about what you're doing.

Peer learning has also been shown to have a positive effect on the learner's clinical reasoning as students are encouraged to reflect on their practice and to openly discuss clinical reasoning approaches together.[15]

Additional benefits to educators have resulted from having more than one student in a practice setting. The majority of educators have reported that by delegating at least 50% of their caseload to students in the collaborative placement model they have had more time to spend facilitating and assessing student learning, supporting junior colleagues and undertaking administrative duties.[9,16] Recent research into different placement models has also enabled utilisation of the whole staff team to be explored.

Promoting a team model of practice education

The team model of practice education is also felt to have potential benefits as a flexible way of delivering education in the practice setting.[10,11] A recent study by Bennett[11] demonstrated that practitioners of all grades have qualities that could play a constructive part in the support of learning within practice learning environments. Findings from the study suggested that junior staff often have a clearer understanding of what it actually feels like to be a student and the involvement of junior staff in placement learning may also promote a climate within the team that supports practice education. A junior colleague would not be expected to take full responsibility for a student in the practice setting but may contribute to the student's learning by reviewing medical notes with a student or engaging in reflective discussion of a case scenario.

> Involving junior grades within the team will help to develop clinical education leaders of the future and could be the key to opening the door for all physiotherapists to accept clinical supervision as part of their role.

If the whole team is involved in the delivery of the placement, learners may gain experience in a variety of situations and from a number of different health professionals. It is also felt that inclusion of more junior staff in the placement enables more experiences from the whole team to be shared, thus promoting reflection on practice[11] A study by Baldry Currens[10] also explored advantages and disadvantages of the team approach. Findings from the study indicated that practice educators welcomed the benefits of this model of practice education, as it felt less intense, allowing them to share responsibility for two students with other team members. Students who experienced the team model also reported benefits from being exposed to different approaches and welcomed the approachability and support gained from working with more junior staff. Baldry Currens[10] also acknowledged the importance of establishing clear lines of communication between all team members in order to prevent students from getting 'mixed messages' relating to diverse treatment approaches or timetabling arrangements. Another essential requirement was the need for educators to ensure that students felt supported within the team, which may at times feel intimidating to a less confident learner.

Whilst the employment of new and flexible models of placement delivery has succeeded in addressing some of the problems related to placement shortages and has had positive educational benefits for both students and practice educators, it has been necessary for higher education institutions (HEIs) and placement providers across health professional groups to explore other ways of promoting team skill development and maximising placement usage. These strategies have included the promotion of Interprofessional Practice Education.

Interprofessional learning opportunities

The importance of developing interprofessional education within university-based and practice-based learning environments has been a prime focus of the

Department of Health document *Working Together, Learning Together.*[17] Interprofessional learning opportunities within practice learning environments are seen to be a key way of preparing students for their future practice in a variety of settings and for working effectively within health professional teams. Whenever possible, opportunities should be arranged for students to spend time with other members of the healthcare team and to learn from students from other professions. These may include attendance at joint case conferences, multidisciplinary team meetings, discharge planning meetings, home visits with other team members and interprofessional student case presentations.[18] Recent developments in health, rehabilitation and social care should enable more interprofessional learning opportunities within the practice learning environment to be explored and developed.[18] For example, the emergence of a growing number of intermediate care settings and community assessment rehabilitation teams within primary care trusts has led to the development of integrated care pathways for patients involving collaboration between all team members. These practice environments potentially offer a range of interprofessional learning opportunities for students on placements, enabling learners from different health professional groups to spend time together assessing patients and engaging in collaborative goal setting. Such activities allow learners to recognise and respect the roles of their colleagues,[19] enabling them to gain more insight into the appropriateness of referrals that they make to other members of the health professional team.

Collaborative strategies supporting practice education

A number of higher education institutions have collaborated to ensure that placement opportunities are optimised. For example, in the South East of England a Physiotherapy Placement Integrated Management System (PPIMS) has been established to facilitate communication between 10 HEIs and placement providers across the Eastern, London and South East regions. Its aim was to provide a one stop communication point for both provider units and educational establishments and to co-ordinate placement offers and uptake and shortages through a common database.

In addition to the placement database, ongoing collaboration between the academic clinical co-ordinators representing the 10 universities within the PPIMS group has led to the formation of common assessment, evaluation and audit tools that have been favourably received by educators and students in the practice setting.

In recent years SHAs, who are now actively engaged in monitoring the quality of placement education, have collaborated with trusts and higher education institutions to develop a range of posts to support uniprofessional and interprofessional practice education within trusts and to increase links between trusts and HEIs. One example is the development of the Practice Placement Facilitator post that has enabled links between trusts and HEIs to be forged and placement capacity and placement learning opportunities to be explored and facilitated.

Practice education networks

The development of practice educator network groups within trusts and across trusts has been an important development in recent years, enabling practice educators to share and discuss issues related to practice education and to gain valuable support from their peers. These networks enable senior practitioners, with the support of their line managers, to take time out from their day-to-day activity in order to reflect on their practice and to explore significant incidents related to practice education with the support of colleagues and on some occasions practice education representatives from their local HEI.

Maintaining the quality of placement learning opportunities

During recent years there has been increased focus on the importance of practice – education placements and the need to assure their quality.[20] The joint NHS and Quality Assurance Agency (QAA) Major Review of all Health Professional Courses has been instigated in order to ensure that the quality of health professional course provision at both pre- and post-registration level meets the required criteria. The QAA[20] emphasise that the quality of placement provision is a shared responsibility between HEIs and the placement providers.

In the future education commissioners and regulators will be implementing OQME (ongoing quality monitoring and evaluation) on an annual basis, in order to ensure that the quality of programmes provided by HEIs and placement providers is maintained between approval of the programme and the initial major review and one major review and the next. The responsibility for meeting the OQME standards rests jointly with the HEI and the practice learning provider.[21] It is therefore essential that collaboration exists between HEIs and placement providers to ensure that the quality of student learning is maintained in both academic and practice environments.

Role development of practice educators

Recognising the ongoing need to support practitioners in developing their educational role within the practice environment to ensure that the quality of practice education meets the standards necessary for supporting practice development, a range of study days and courses have been developed across health professional groups. These include a range of uniprofessional and interprofessional study days based in HEIs or on trust sites that focus on broad aspects of education exploring the role of the practice educator and ways of planning, facilitating and assessing student learning in the practice environment. A number of HEIs also offer practice educators a range of Master's level modules and programme routes focusing on practice education that are delivered on campus, or in some cases offered through distance learning mode, including online delivery.

Accreditation of educators in the practice setting

The Chartered Society of Physiotherapy's ACE (Accreditation of Clinical Educators) scheme was launched in March 2004. The scheme was designed to give educators in the practice setting more support and recognition in their role as clinical educators. The scheme has clear links with practitioners' overall continuing professional development (CPD) activity, as a large proportion of the evidence that practice educators gather to meet the ACE learning outcomes may also be used to contribute to their CPD portfolio of evidence for re-registration purposes.

The introduction of the ACE scheme has provided an opportunity for educators in the practice setting to gain recognition of their professional status as practice educators and has been designed and developed by the CSP to recognise the valuable role played by practice educators and to raise the quality of clinical education throughout the UK.

Practice educators are encouraged to view the ACE scheme as an opportunity and not a mandatory requirement and it is hoped that in due course practice educators will aspire to achieve accredited status.

Practice educators wishing to achieve accredited status may pursue either a programme (taught) route or an experiential (profile development) route in order to demonstrate evidence of their achievement of six learning outcomes. The learning outcomes focus on the educator's ability to:

- describe the role and attributes of the effective clinical educator
- apply learning theories that are appropriate for adult and professional learners
- plan, implement and facilitate learning in the clinical setting
- apply sound principles and judgement in the assessment of performance in the clinical setting
- evaluate the learning experience
- reflect on experience and formulate action plans to improve future practice.

The scheme is felt to be 'central to the delivery of quality education in the practice environment'[22] and to link closely with the continuing professional development and the NHS and Quality Assurance Agency's reviews.

Although the ACE scheme was initially designed for physiotherapy educators, its potential has been recognised by other health professional groups. The six learning outcomes of the ACE scheme have recently been adopted by the Council of Occupational Therapists (COT) and will form the basis of the APPLE scheme (Accreditation of Practice Placement Educators).

In addition, other healthcare professions are currently considering adopting a derivative of the ACE scheme.

Managing placement learning within trusts

Fostering a climate of learning within your practice setting

The Department of Health[17] published an influential document *Working Together, Learning Together: a framework for lifelong learning for the NHS*, which set out a vision and comprehensive strategy for lifelong learning.

The emphasis within the framework is on the provision of a learning infrastructure that is accessible in terms of time and location, fostering exchange of information, team working and promoting a community of learning. This vision for a community of learning is closely linked with the need to provide an effective learning environment for any student in the practice setting that enables them to feel supported, promoting an exchange of ideas between the educator and learner and valuing the learner's contribution to the learning process.[23]

Although this chapter has focused primarily on current issues related to student learning, within individual trusts there will be a range of educator/learner interactions that individual practitioners may regularly be involved in. The list of learners may include pre- and post-registration learners from across the health professions, care assistants, rehabilitation assistants, those returning to the profession, patients and carers.[3] All educational activities can benefit a practice setting as they provide valuable opportunities for:

1 Continuing professional development.[22]
2 Development of organisational skills.[24]
3 Reflection and sharing of knowledge.[25]
4 Evaluation of practice.[3]
5 Interprofessional working[18] and team skill development.[10,11]

It may be worth considering the implications of the introduction of the NHS Knowledge and Skills Framework[26] linked to the Agenda for Change pay gateways. This framework outlines a number of core dimensions of professional practice. Review of the core dimensions indicates that they embrace a number of skills that are clearly linked to education in the practice setting. One of the general core dimensions of the Knowledge and Skills Framework (KSF) focuses on Learning and Development and highlights a range of ways by which practitioners can develop their knowledge and skills in relation to this core dimension. Active engagement in practice education will therefore offer practitioners at all stages in their professional development the opportunity to develop their educational skills within the KSF framework.

In order to ensure that the quality of these learning and teaching opportunities within the practice setting is optimised it is essential that practice educators receive support and encouragement from their managers to prevent practice education from being seen as a secondary activity. Examples of good practice exist across health professional groups when managers are actively engaged in the promotion of practice education and have a clear vision of their trust's placement capacity and the quality of the environment that should support placement learning. Such practice often has a positive impact on recruitment, as students often seek staff posts where they have had positive placements.

Although guidelines for supporting placement learning identify criteria that managers should fulfil in relation to education in the practice setting,[27] findings from a study by Baldry Currens[6] indicated that some managers remained unaware of the activities within their department that related to clinical education. As a result senior practitioners felt that their managers did not always fully appreciate the complexity of their role as practice educators. This apparent lack of interest from managers resulted in practice educators feeling unsupported in their role. The perceptions of educators in the study were substantiated by comments from managers that suggest that practice education was not one of their prime concerns. Difficulties also arose when decisions regarding placement offers were delegated to individual practitioners, resulting in a lack of overview in relation to placement capacity. It must be noted, however, that this was a relatively small-scale study and only five pairs of managers from one education consortium were interviewed.

In contrast, managers interviewed for a study by Crouch *et al*[24] that explored 1:1; 2:1 and 3:1 placements across occupational therapy and physiotherapy fully acknowledged the importance of supporting practice education, suggesting that the more students that came through their trusts on placement, the better it was for them in terms of recruitment.

Two health professional case studies that formed part of a recent audit undertaken as part of a higher education funded (HEFCE) national project, Making Practice-based Learning Work, also indicate that support from managers and other team members and acknowledgement of the importance of student education remain key requirements for the success of student learning in the practice setting.[28,29]

Box 4.1 Top ten tips for managers – supporting practice education

1 Ensure practice educators have access to appropriate preparation courses.
2 Ensure students/learners are made to feel part of the department.
3 Promote learning by creating a positive environment for learning within the workplace.[3]
4 Pay attention to the possible constraints on learning.
5 Encourage the creative use of different models of practice education.[7,11]
6 Ensure that those with practice education skills feed into learning opportunities for all staff.
7 Encourage practice educators to use their transferable skills in patient education and educational sessions provided for other health professionals.
8 Foster a positive attitude within your practice environment to support accreditation of educators, for example ACE & APPLE schemes for practice educators.
9 Think of the provision of high-quality practice education as a selling and marketing point for your NHS trust and of importance in recruitment and retention.
10 Capitalise on learner feedback following their practice education experience in your trust and use these to fully develop the quality of the practice education offered.

Supporting individual learning experiences

This chapter has initially explored the 'bigger picture' of practice education and has considered national issues impacting on the provision of practice learning opportunities, together with opportunities for practice education that exist within individual trusts. A model of practice education that can be employed by educators to support individual learning experiences is introduced and explored.

The learning experience model in action

A model of placement learning that follows a typical curriculum development cycle proposed by Moore *et al*[3] provides a framework for a total learning

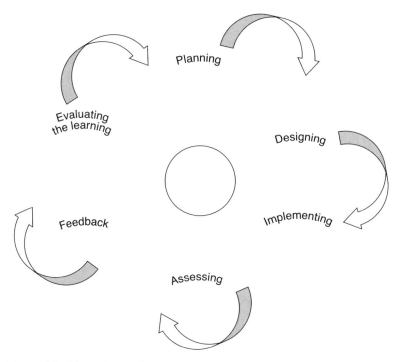

Figure 4.1 Model of learning in the practice setting

experience for a learner or group of learners. The model has six stages that can be employed to support learning in the practice setting.

Each stage of the model is considered in turn.

- **Planning the learning:** During the planning phase of the model the educator needs to consider the learner's stage of education, the HEI's course requirements and the placement pattern and duration. It is useful if the whole team prepares in advance and agrees plans for welcoming and inducting the learner into the department. This phase of the cycle enables educators to plan a draft timetable outlining learning opportunities and feedback meetings, enabling other health professionals who may be contributing to the learning to plan in advance.
- **Designing the learning:** During the design phase of the learning the educator and learner should negotiate a learning agreement or learning contract that takes into account the individual needs of the learner and their preferred learning style. This example of good practice enables learning resources to be identified by both parties, and feedback times to be agreed, together with methods for assessing and evaluating the learning outcomes. It is essential that educators consider the learner's background, as mature students may have very different learning needs to students who have entered a health professional course directly from school.
- **Implementing the learning:** During the implementation stage practice educators should employ a range of learning and teaching strategies to facilitate the learning. Practice educators should ensure that a range of uniprofessional and interprofessional learning opportunities are promoted that enable the student

to develop skills in communication, clinical reasoning, assessment, treatment management and team work. Whenever possible adult learning approaches[30] should be promoted that encourage learners to be independent and self-directed in their learning, demonstrating their ability to reflect on and evaluate the effectiveness of their practice.

- **Assessing and providing feedback on the learning:** It is essential for educators who are engaged in the assessment of students in the practice setting to consider the learner's stage of learning and to link the assessment to the learning outcomes of the placement together with the guidelines for assessment and the assessment criteria. The majority of assessment methods used by educators in the practice setting include observation and questioning approaches. Assessment of learning should be fair and reliable but should avoid giving students who are weak the benefit of the doubt as ultimately standards will be lowered and patient care may be compromised.[31] Feedback should enable the student to have a clear understanding about their progress in the practice setting and should be delivered at regular intervals in a private area and should provide the learner with clear guidance to enable them to meet their learning outcomes.

- **Evaluating the learning:** Evaluation of any learning experience is essential to ensure that the effectiveness of the learning and teaching approaches is explored and the quality of the learning is established. Evaluation is usually an empowering process as it allows both educators and learners to reflect on both the positive and negative aspects of any learning experience and to consider areas for future development. As educators in the practice setting you may wish to use the evaluation forms currently used by your local education provider or you may consider designing your own local evaluation form in conjunction with your learners and other colleagues.

The checklist below (*see* Box 4.2) has been designed to provide educators who are engaged in supporting learners in the practice setting with some key points of reference that are suitable for use with any learner at any stage of education.

Box 4.2 Checklist of good practice for practice educators

1 Planning the learning
- Consider the model of practice education.
- Plan induction period and consider resources including other team members.
- Prepare a draft timetable.

2 Design learning
- Assess the learner's needs.
- Take into account the learner's preferred learning style.
- Negotiate a learning contract.
- Adapt the programme to meet the learner's needs.

3 Implementing the learning
- Develop open communication with the learner.
- Facilitate the learning using a variety of learning and teaching approaches.[3,32]

- Observe good practice in relation to feedback, providing the learner with regular constructive feedback and allowing time for discussion within a supportive environment.

4 Assessing the learning
   - Organise assessment opportunities.
   - Observe the learner and allow time for building up an accurate impression of their performance.
   - Adopt an encouraging manner when questioning.
   - Adhere to criteria and assessment guidelines.
   - Encourage learners to evaluate their performance.

5 Feedback
   - Provide feedback that identifies strengths and areas for development.
   - Sandwich constructive criticism with positive aspects of the learner's performance.
   - Encourage two-way feedback and peer feedback.
   - Ensure feedback is delivered in a private area.

6 Evaluate the learning from different perspectives
   - The learner/learners.
   - The department.
   - Professional colleagues.
   - Learn from the evaluation and feed the evaluation findings into the next educational event.

Conclusion

The issues discussed and the range of models presented in this chapter may in some small way contribute to the ongoing debate related to the management of practice education, which by its very nature continues to provide both challenges and rewards for all engaged in its delivery, and ongoing quality monitoring of its effectiveness. However, in recent years it has been encouraging to note that there has been an increased focus on the need to ensure that practice educators are given recognition for their vital contribution to the professional development of future health professionals. It is therefore essential that all parties involved in the organisation of education in the practice setting actively collaborate to ensure that practice educators receive the support necessary to provide high-quality learning experiences that continue to be both rich and stimulating for both learners and educators.

References

1 College of Occupational Therapists. *College of Occupational Therapists' Standards for Education: pre-registration education standards*. London: COT; 2003.
2 Chartered Society of Physiotherapy. *Curriculum Framework for Qualifying Programmes in Physiotherapy*. London: CSP; 2002.
3 Moore A, Hilton R, Morris J *et al*. *The Clinical Educator Role Development: a self-directed learning text*. Edinburgh: Churchill Livingstone; 1997.

4 Department of Health. *The NHS Plan: a plan for investment, a plan for reform*. London: Stationery Office; 2000.

5 Martin M, Morris J, Moore A *et al*. Evaluating practice education models in Occupational Therapy: comparing 1:1, 2:1 and 3:1 placements. *British Journal of Occupational Therapy*. 2004. **67**(5): 192–200.

6 Baldry Currens JA, Bithell CP. Clinical education: listening to different perspectives. *Physiotherapy*. 2000. **86**(12): 645–53.

7 Moore A, Morris J, Crouch V *et al*. Evaluation of physiotherapy clinical education comparing 1:2, 2:1 and 3:1 models. *Physiotherapy*. 2003. **89**: 489–501.

8 Huddleston R. Clinical placements for the Professions Allied to Medicine. Part 2. Placement shortages? Two models that can solve the problem. *British Journal of Occupational Therapy*. 1999. **62**(7): 295–8.

9 Baldry Currens J, Bithell C. The 2:1 clinical placement model – perceptions of clinical educators and students. *Physiotherapy*. 2003. **89**(4): 203–64.

10 Baldry Currens J. *An evaluation of three clinical placement models for undergraduate physiotherapy students. Report on Phase 11 of the Clinical Education Project*. University of East London; 2000.

11 Bennett R. Clinical education. Perceived abilities/qualities of clinical educators and team supervision of students. *Physiotherapy*. 2003. **89**(7): 432–42.

12 Lloyd J, Baldry J, Currens J. Changing the one to one clinical placement model. *Physiotherapy Frontline*. 2000. **January 15**: 15.

13 Ladyshewsky R. Peer assisted learning in clinical education: a review of the terms and learning principles. *Journal of Physical Therapy Education*. 2000. **14**(2): 15–22.

14 Lincoln M, McAllister LL. Facilitating peer learning in clinical education. *Medical Teacher*. 1993. **15**(1): 17–25.

15 Ladyshewsky R. The impact of peer coaching on the clinical reasoning of the novice practitioner. *Physiotherapy Canada*. 2004. **56**(1): 15–26.

16 Ladyshewsky R. Enhancing service productivity in acute inpatient service settings using a collaborative clinical education model. *Physical Therapy*. 1995. **75**(2): 503–10.

17 Department of Health. *Working Together, Learning Together: a framework for lifelong learning in the NHS*. London: Department of Health; 2001.

18 Hilton R, Morris J. Student placements – is there evidence supporting team skill development in practice settings? *Journal of Interprofessional Care*. 2001. **15**(2): 171–83.

19 Green RJ, Cavell GF, Jackson SHD. Interprofessional clinical education of medical and pharmacy student. *Medical Education*. 1996. **30**: 129–33.

20 Quality Assurance Agency for Higher Education. *Code of Practice for the Assurance of Academic Quality and Standards in Higher Education: placement learning*. Gloucester: QAA; 2001.

21 Quality Assurance Agency. *Prototype document for Approval and Ongoing Quality Monitoring and Enhancement (OQME)*. Gloucester: QAA; 2004.

22 Pope G. CSP raises clinical standards with ACE scheme. News release. The Chartered Society of Physiotherapy. London: CSP Communications and Marketing; 2004.

23 Lickman P, Simms L, Greene C. Learning environment: the catalyst for work excitement. *Journal of Continuing Education in Nursing*. 1993. **17**: 682–91.

24 Crouch V, Moore A, Morris J *et al*. *An Evaluation of Clinical Education Models for Occupational Therapy and Physiotherapy: comparing 1:1, 2:1 and 3:1 placement models*. Brighton: University of Brighton. 2001.

25 Clouder L. Reflective practice: realising its potential. *Physiotherapy*. 2002. **86**(10): 517–19.

26 Department of Health. *Knowledge and Skills Framework*. London: DOH; 2004.

27 Chartered Society of Physiotherapy. *Clinical Education Placement Guidelines*. London: CSP; 2003.

28 Dawson P. *Physiotherapy Case Study Report. An overview of the nature of the preparation of*

practice educators in five health care disciplines. Making practice-based learning work. 2004. www.practicebasedlearning.org.

29 McClure P. *Occupational Therapy Case Study Report. An overview of the nature of the preparation of practice educators in five health care disciplines. Making practice-based learning work.* 2004. www.practicebasedlearning.org.

30 Knowles M, Holton E, Swanson R. *The Adult Learner.* 5th ed. Houston: Gulf Publishing Company; 1998.

31 Ilott I, Murphy R. *Success and Failure in Professional Education: assessing the evidence.* London: Whurr; 1999.

32 McAllister L, Lincoln M. *Methods in Speech and Language Pathology Series.* Clinical Education in Speech – Language Pathology. London: Whurr; 2004.

Chapter 5

Work-based learning

Jonathan Burton and Neil Jackson

Work-based learning in the NHS

The needs of patients and local communities are paramount in the new NHS and must be supported by an appropriate system of planning, educating and developing a multiprofessional/multidisciplinary workforce of healthcare professionals at national and local levels. Along with modernisation in the NHS comes a greater need for lifelong learning to ensure that NHS staff continue to develop and enhance their knowledge and skills throughout their working lives.[1]

Work-based learning as a model of lifelong learning enables healthcare professionals working as individuals and in teams in the NHS to participate in regular and systematic educational activity. This in turn will contribute to the maintenance and development of clinical competence and performance and promote quality service provision for patients. When applied effectively, work-based learning will also raise staff morale and increase their sense of purpose, while enhancing job satisfaction and retention in the NHS workforce.

In this chapter, we will look at what happens to individuals working in the health service. The most typical career for a health professional will consist of a period of pre-registration education and training, with qualification in his/her early twenties, followed by a potential career of 30, 40 or even more years. So as we write this chapter, those qualifying in 2006 might still be working as professionals in a 'health service' in 2050.

There are less typical careers, or work patterns, and these are likely to become more common. Unskilled entrants into the workforce, or individuals who have had other basic training, can be offered ways of retraining so that they too can take on skilled tasks in healthcare. In a way, such individuals are simply entering the workforce with a newly achieved set of skills at an older age. The completion of basic training (also known as pre-qualification training), whether that happens at the age of 21 or 31 or 51, represents the end of the beginning of learning for the individual worker. What happens thereafter, over a working life of several years or several decades, is an evolutionary process in which work-based learning has a very important role. The basic training with which we enter the workforce is merely a preparation and cannot ensure on its own that individual workers will remain appropriately skilled for their changing roles in a changing world. If we learn well and if we work in teams which learn well, then it follows that the work that we do will be better. Learning and working are intertwined. As David Boud[2] says:

> The defining characteristic of work-based learning is that working and learning are coincident. Learning tasks are influenced by the nature of

work and, in turn, work is influenced by the nature of the learning that occurs.

In this chapter, we look broadly at work-based learning as it applies to the health service. But first we must start with some definitions. What is work-based learning?

Definitions of work-based learning

In the literature, work-based learning is also known as workplace based learning. We find the latter term rather restrictive as it does not embrace the idea that much work-based learning actually takes place away from the workplace.

Seagraves et al[3] offer a useful definition of work-based learning as learning that takes place at, for or from work – in other words, it takes place geographically at our workplace, purposefully for improving our work performance or causally from our experience of work. You will, perhaps, understand these three concepts more easily by interpreting them through the fictional vignette (see Box 5.2) that is set out later in this chapter.

One of the problems with Seagraves' definition of work-based learning is that it does not emphasise strongly enough the fact that work-based learning takes place both at work and away from work. A second definition, therefore, which you might find useful, is that of Hugh Barr.[4] He differentiates between work-located learning (that which occurs geographically at work) and work-related learning (that which occurs away from work but whose focus is the process of work.) His emphasis here is that the learning, wherever it takes place, is undertaken with the primary purpose of doing the work better. A common theme, then, in the definitions of work-based learning is that they describe a situation where, in Boud's words, 'learning tasks are influenced by the nature of work'. For this reason, many authors do see the growing interest in work-based learning as coming from an economically and managerially driven view of the purpose of learning. They say that work-based learning has been promoted for economic reasons, as a tool to make a more efficient or more competitive workforce. For example, Brennan and Little[5] wrote in 1996 that:

> The education system has been urged to ensure that people are given an effective foundation for working life and are motivated to achieve their potential, to take more responsibility for their own development, and to continue to develop the skills that they, and their employers, need.

From these economically based arguments, it will follow that the primary imperative for the workforce is to earn a living by contributing in a certain, often prescribed, way to society's activities. Education and training and, *ipso facto*, work-based learning can become instruments to increase the productivity and effectiveness of the workforce.

From the individual person's point of view, of course, there will be other imperatives for their working lives, such as the need to derive satisfaction from a job, and enjoy the society of work colleagues and so on. In the same way, it is possible to counterbalance the strictly utilitarian view of work-based learning and see it more for what it means for individuals and teams and how it is experienced. There should be the recognition that 'it happens anyway':[6] it is a natural, human response to the experience of work. As such, it should be better understood as should its benefits.

Who is involved in work-based learning and how are they involved?

Both teams and individuals are involved in work-based learning. We should not forget the patient here, as he or she is not only the focus of care, but is also the agent of work-based learning. What happens to patients or should happen to them is a major focus of learning and, as we will show in the next section, it is the experience of working with patients that can provide so much material for learning.

Learning will take place as a reaction to what is going on at work, and, if the worker is a nurse or an AHP, 'what is going on at work' means, primarily, having contact with patients. The learning reaction to daily work may be subject to certain refinements (such as the process of self-reflection or the input of a supervising colleague). However, the actual 'drama of work' is to an extent unplanned. The idea that we learn from experience is not new. Aristotle addressed it when he wrote about practical wisdom. Knowles, Kolb, Schön and Eraut have written about what kind of knowledge is learned from experience and how it can be supported. The contrary argument – that we do not necessarily learn from experience – has been put forward by Saul Alinsky.[7] If significant learning is to occur on the basis of experience, then it will happen when experiences are reflected upon, patterns recognised and synthesised.

A wealth of previous work-based experience is said to give rise to tacit knowledge. Tacit knowledge is practical and experience based, is not written down systematically, and is said to help people in knowing 'how' to do something. The other sort of knowledge is explicit. This form of knowledge is articulated and written down, and is learned so that people know 'what' to do.

Scientific knowledge (or explicit knowledge) informs practice and is the basis of professional practice. Experience of practice leads to tacit knowledge and tacit knowledge is acquired through exposure to the work situation.

Another concept to understand is that of incremental learning. Healthcare workers adapt to the changes in scientific knowledge, often without going on taught courses, and most of this adaptation comes from incremental learning.[8] Incremental learning, for example through reading, e-learning, collaborative learning, and attending short updates, will help to expand the basic scientific knowledge or explicit knowledge which came with qualification. However, it is not possible to build up the capacity of the healthcare workforce purely on the basis of incremental learning. New skills and competencies have also to be learned through formal teaching. We will now go on to discuss the concept of the 'skills escalator' in the generation of a more skilled workforce and the role of work-based learning within this whole area. Our next discussion is about primary care, but might equally apply to the acute sector.

Within the NHS, the 'skills escalator' is the term given by the NHS to the strategy developed to increase and change the workforce. Bowler describes the 'skills escalator' in the NHS as follows:[9]

> The essence of this approach is that staff are encouraged through a strategy of lifelong learning to constantly renew and extend their skills and knowledge, enabling them to move up the escalator. Meanwhile, efficiencies and skill mix benefits are generated by delegating roles, work and responsibilities down the escalator where appropriate.

There are a number of educational methods by which the skills escalator can be made real, and a significant amount of these will be work-based learning. The intention is that members of staff are encouraged through lifelong learning to renew and extend their skills and knowledge to the extent of their ability so they can move up the escalator. Meanwhile efficiencies and skill mix benefits are generated through changing roles, with elements of work or responsibility passing to the most appropriate staff.

Reviewing current initiatives to develop the primary care workforce along the 'escalator' model suggests four main transition points.

1 Untrained people being brought in to work in administrative or supporting roles (e.g. training for receptionists).
2 Existing non-clinical staff taking on new roles and responsibilities; these may be clinical, e.g. healthcare assistant (HCA), or managerial, e.g. within primary care, practice management. Staff could be recruited from outside the NHS for these roles too.
3 Developing professional roles: professionals with special interests such as nurse practitioners and clinical specialist AHPs.
4 Developing the general practitioner (GP) role: GPs with special interests.

There are other examples of primary care team members escalating their skills (for example, Practice Manager plus – where a non-clinical manager takes on management roles more usually carried out by a GP in the practice) but these four broad sections cover the majority of role enhancement. It is worth pointing out that these developments are linked: for example, the broadening of the administrative staff roles to include some routine clinical duties frees up a practice nurse for specialist activities.

Individuals who are learning new skills in the way described above will almost always be exposed to structured work-based learning as part of their courses. The work-based learning may include academically accredited work-based learning projects, attachments, apprenticeships, work-related assessments and appraisals, work-based tutorials and one-on-one and peer supervision based on their clinical work.

The three dimensions of work-based learning

We have already explained how work-based learning embraces learning experiences as diverse as experiential learning and formal retraining. So it is clear that work-based learning can mean different things to different people, a difference which is largely conditioned by settings and contexts.[10,11] To a university department which is involved in supplying specific educational opportunities to the NHS, work-based learning will have a particular meaning. To an AHP who is having his/her case work supervised, work-based learning will mean something completely different. The university lecturer and the AHP in practice will have their own understanding of what is important in work-based learning, reflecting different learning cultures, organisational structures and desired outcomes. We propose three dimensions of work-based learning (*see* Box 5.1).

Box 5.1 Three dimensions of work-based learning

1 accredited work-based learning as part of university-based course (degree or otherwise)
2 work-based learning as part of a managed and structured occupational learning programme, which is obligatory or highly recommended for certain jobs
3 work-based learning as an individual and/or collective responsibility within a work setting

---

Whilst the first two dimensions of work-based learning are structured, involve formal learning and are part of a managed approach to developing new skills, the third dimension is essentially a form of self-directed learning.

We will illustrate these three dimensions of work-based learning by giving three examples.

For some individuals, accredited work-based learning as part of a university-based course may provide opportunities for developing new skills and may open up new horizons, both personally and professionally. For example, it has been described how a group of nurses undertook a modular, work-based learning programme. There was input from a local university and the students learned to perform literature searches, plan healthcare interventions based on the literature, and introduce changes to practice – in a way which they had not been able to do previously.

An example of work-based learning as part of a managed and structured occupational learning programme, which is obligatory or highly recommended for certain jobs, can be found in the training provided by NHS 24. NHS 24 is a Scottish telephone advice service for the general public and is staffed by advisors who have a general nursing background. The advisors need to be trained to work on the phone and follow computer-based algorithms. The programme of preparatory and continuing learning has been designed to prepare them for the realities of their jobs. It uses simulations, feedback, preceptorship and other sorts of work-related learning.[12]

Finally, there is the work-based learning which is largely self-directed and relatively unstructured. Frequently, it occurs on the basis of previously established professional capability and is essentially incremental. Incremental learning has been discussed earlier in the chapter. Learning by doing the job is essential for those whose practice is independent, for example GPs and community occupational therapists. Simulations and theory prepare but do not substitute for the real thing, where a practitioner must decide autonomously what to do and take responsibility for that judgement.

A vignette that is fictional illustrates some aspects of this third dimension of work-based learning. Anne is an imaginary person, and you may cast her in your own mind as a technically competent, highly trained, conscientious but slightly inexperienced physiotherapist, perhaps a few years out of training. The inspiration for this vignette is Mark Cole's[13] account of the portfolio-based learning undertaken by physiotherapists. The story of Anne's learning shows that her learning has been occasioned by her own curiosity and discomfort at not knowing.

Box 5.2 Vignette 1

Anne is a physiotherapist. She works in a community hospital, in a department with one other physiotherapist and one physiotherapy assistant. She is employed by the local community trust. She is dealing with a patient who has been referred with a strained calf muscle, acquired during sporting activity, and which is making further sporting activity almost impossible. The patient asks her how long he must expect to be 'off sports' with this injury, as he is making a claim on an insurance policy, but she does not feel confident to give an opinion. She asks her more experienced colleague, who quotes some published works, and on the basis of these she is able to give the patient some evidence-based information. This is an example of learning at work.

Anne keeps a learning portfolio for her own continuing professional development and she records this learning episode in her portfolio. She attends a peer learning group once a quarter at which group members discuss their own portfolios. Anne shares this learning episode with colleagues, and there is a general discussion about what to do if you 'don't know the answer'. Anne realises that everyone has this problem (not knowing the answer) on a regular basis and finds it reassuring to know that this is part and parcel of professional practice. This realisation, and the discussion on which it was based, is an example of learning from work. Anne realises that some of the colleagues in the group are much more confident in getting answers to such problems than she is, and especially those who are adept at doing internet searches. How could she improve her skills at using the internet to do searches?

She could sit in with a colleague who is adept at such things. Or she might seek out a specific course. Through either approach she would expect to improve her skills. Soon, she will find that she can use the desktop at work to do quick searches, sometimes telling patients that she will look things up and tell them the answer at their next appointment, or even whilst they are present. This last bit of learning – learning to do the internet searches – is an example of work-based learning: in this case it is an example of learning for work.

Assessment of work-based learning

There are many ways of assessing work-based learning or the effectiveness of the learning environment and these have been summarised in respect of primary care.[14] Some may say that self-directed learning, as set out in the example of Anne above, is too chancy and that a health service cannot be allowed to run on such a haphazard system of learning. This argument, however, is based on the premise that individuals will only learn if they are taught. A retrospective learning audit may help to dispel the general pessimism that underlies this argument and help to show that learning has been effective and how it has been effective. Vignette 2 (*see* Box 5.3) illustrates such a retrospective learning audit.

Box 5.3 Vignette 2

Of 18 experienced GPs, only three had ever been on a course about heart failure, since qualifying as GPs. Heart failure is a common condition seen in primary care. In a discussion seminar, all 18 demonstrated a reasonable understanding of the recently released National Institute of Clinical Excellence (NICE) guidelines on the management of chronic heart failure,[15] thereby showing that they had successfully updated their knowledge of heart failure since they had qualified. During a facilitated discussion, they were able to identify the myriad ways in which this incremental learning had occurred, for example via their own personal study, their experience with patients, what they had learned from colleagues and so on.

There have been many attempts to encourage professionals to formalise and stimulate this essentially informal approach to learning, for example by encouraging the use of portfolios as evidence of learning achieved.[16]

Failures do occur, however, and it is important to be aware of these. The learning environment may be at fault or the individual learner may simply be unaware that his or her practice is inappropriate or out of date.[17]

In the present approach to continuing professional development (CPD) for all professional groups there should be some safeguards to ensure that there has been an appropriate degree of assessment of professional practice – whether it be by self-assessment, peer assessment or third party assessment.[18] For a fuller account of the connection between assessment and work-based learning, readers should refer to our chapter in *Work Based Learning in Primary Care*.[19] At present there is much public debate as to the practicalities of assessment and how assessment might ensure patient safety and best practice.

Learning, experience and accountability

In speaking about learning, experience and accountability we need to have an understanding of how everyday experiences shape professional judgement and practice. It is this reality that makes the learner centredness of education critical. Whatever the environment, learning begins with the individual and their own experiences, as the vignette about Anne earlier in this chapter showed. Learning must be contemporary, taking account of present realities and present experiences.

Sometimes what we do at work and what we need to learn to do this work seem to be out of kilter with the major interests of the health service – its policies, its views of good practice and its managerialism driven by the need for accountability. At other times what we do at work, and our learning, are comfortably in touch with current directions of a managed health service. Healthcare workers need to develop a sophisticated approach to learning. They need to see that their own interests and those of the health service have to be finely balanced. Learning has to occur in a way which is sensitive to the demands of external reality. Professional practice and professional learning have always been located within the discipline of such accountability. We choose the word 'discipline' deliberately and discriminate between the concept of discipline (which is under the influence of self) and the concept of control (which is under the influence of others). In an ideal world, everyone would have developed the discipline to learn from experience, though not everyone does so, nor does everyone learn effectively. There will be learning failures and systems need to be developed to identify and remedy these.

Notwithstanding these problems, learning must not be judged solely by its problems (although such judgements do have to be made). There needs also to be a generous understanding that takes into account the great volume of learning that leads to appropriate outcomes despite the external demands on the workforce.

Promoting and understanding effective learning

Over a lifetime (that is what lifelong learning is about), learners should have it within their grasp to devise systems of personal and collaborative learning which are appropriate for their working situations and which can become appropriately rigorous. But does this happen and does it happen over the long term? Characteristics of self-directed learning, common among several professional groups in primary care, suggest that work-based learning forms a critical part of the professional passage from novice to retirement.[20] In our previous published work we have written about the world of nurses, GPs and practice managers.[21] Anne McKee and Michael Watts have shown how practice teams are capable of becoming competent in self-directed learning.[22]

We have shown how for many individuals and teams the culture of self-deliberation is strong enough to enable successful, team-based and self-directed learning to occur. It is something about resting responsibility for learning on those who are already carrying through wide-ranging responsibilities in their adult and working lives. It is the opposite of expecting learners to fail and reflects a liberal educational philosophy articulated by Dewey in the United States of America and Stenhouse in the United Kingdom.[23,24]

For each of us, the context of work changes with time. External changes such as those associated with the advances of science, the development of the role of healthcare, consumerism, evidence-based practice and professional account-ability all demand further adaptations. The science behind healthcare and the practice of healthcare become context (workplace) bound. Without 'going with the flow' health professionals would be hopelessly at sea within a few years of independent practice.

The challenges for work-based learning

We see two major challenges for work-based learning. The first is to identify the added value, which could flow from attempts to make work-based learning disciplined and rigorous. This is about asking the best questions about what we are doing at work.[21] These questions must be sensitive to the unique context of professional or occupational learning.

The second challenge is to understand the balance between the three dimensions of work-based learning (*see* Box 5.1) and how each of these prepares us for practice. How important is the freedom to learn inherent in self-directed learning? Who is most likely to benefit from a university-based modular programme? How important are structured programmes? Which dimensions of work-based learning make us capable and competent in the long term? Do workers from different professional groups have different needs and expectations in this respect – for example, GPs, community physiotherapists and primary care nurses? How do learners experience a chain of learning and adaptation experiences, which go to create competent self-directed learning – and, again, are there differences according to professional and educational backgrounds? Much has yet to be learned about work-based learning.

Who should decide what is learned?

A liberal approach to the value of learning has to accommodate itself to our regulated society. It can continue to exist as long as the health service and its workers give a service which is safe and evidence based and patients are well served. For this reason, learning will continue to be informed by the need for accountability.

There are many stakeholders in the educational process: patients, employers and workers. In limiting the educational process to the perspective of employers alone, there is the real risk that education will become captive to short-term visions of instant need on the smaller scale and political visions of economic need on the larger scale.[25] We have already written about the problems that stem from too narrow a view of what should be learned.[26]

Some occupations and professions have more freedom to learn than others, and in the concept of the three dimensions of work-based learning, it is clear that, in many situations, learning is obligatory or highly recommended before certain types of work can be done. In these situations the worker is not free to learn if he or she wants to work. In professions where there is more traditional freedom for learning, for example those where independent practice is achieved after initial training, there is only freedom if there is also responsibility. In other words, there is a contract between the individual and those he or she serves, which expresses the parameters within which that freedom exists. The freedom is qualified by the willingness to serve – 'in service is perfect freedom'.[27] This is an admission that what is done by the individual is defined by external influences, although the individual has choice as to how he or she prepares him/herself to respond to those influences.

If we go back to one of the examples we have quoted earlier in this chapter, that of the nurse advisors working for NHS 24, then it is clear that these nurses appear to have relatively little freedom to make judgements. They give advice almost entirely according to a computer-generated protocol. They do not go to work with the responsibility for making independent judgements, but serve the health service in another – very important – way. On the other hand, the GPs who showed that they were *au fait* with the new guidelines for managing chronic heart failure had shown how they had been effective self-directed learners.

What does all this mean? It means that, for some, work-based learning is about getting equipped for a job in which personal judgement is perhaps less important than following procedures, though even for those who follow procedures, it remains important that they can think critically and act responsibly. For others, there are high levels of responsibility and the need to make decisions in a wide range of situations. The podiatrist, the physiotherapist and the GP have different and changing clinical roles. What is that difference and how are their roles changing in practice? At what points in their career do they need to learn differently for those roles and when might shared work-based learning be appropriate?

It appears that as healthcare workers move upwards in their careers, it becomes more important for them to develop as independent learners. Work-based learning can help them prepare for this greater independence. The strength of the modularised university courses in work-based learning is that they help students to develop independence in practice and learning, first by learning how to learn and then by learning how to have influence at work. For each of the situations that we have discussed there is an appropriate model of work-based learning and, if not, the opportunity to devise one.

Work-based learning. A model of lifelong learning in the NHS

In the pursuit of lifelong learning in the NHS, models of education and development are required to give NHS staff a clear understanding of how their own roles integrate with those of others in the healthcare system. In addition, the emphasis on delivering quality standards in the NHS has been frequently highlighted within its various policy documents, for example *A First Class Service: quality in the new NHS*.[28] To deliver the quality agenda in the NHS, lifelong learning for all healthcare professionals is required to meet the challenge of a fast-changing world, medical advances, new technologies and new approaches to patient care. Work-based learning as a model of lifelong learning in the NHS can contribute towards delivering the quality agenda and provide benefits for employers, employees (possibly also enhancing their retention and development in the workforce) and patients in the NHS. These benefits include the promotion of individual and team development within NHS organisations; the enhancement of self-motivation, critical thinking and reflective practice; a greater understanding of working within the complex environment of the new NHS; and enabling a balance to be achieved between personal fulfilment for individual healthcare professionals and the wider needs of the employing organisation and the NHS as a whole.

References

1 Jackson N. Work based learning and the retention and development of the NHS workforce *Work Based Learning in Primary Care*. 2003; 1: 5–10.
2 Boud D. Knowledge at work: issues of learning. In: Boud D, Solomon N, editors. *Work-based Learning. A new higher education*. Buckingham: Open University Press, 2001.
3 Seagraves L, Osborne M, Neal P *et al. Learning in Smaller Companies*. Final report. Stirling: University of Stirling, 1996.

4 Barr H. Interprofessional issues and work based learning. In: Burton J, Jackson N, editors. *Work Based Learning in Primary Care*. Abingdon: Radcliffe Medical Press, 2003.

5 Brennan J, Little B. *A Review of Work Based Learning in Higher Education*. Sheffield: Department of Education and Employment, 1996.

6 Burton J, Jackson N. *Work Based Learning in Primary Care*. Abingdon: Radcliffe Medical Press, 2003.

7 Alinsky SD. *Rules for Radicals*. New York: Random House, 1972.

8 Eraut, M, Alderton J, Cole, G *et al*. Learning from other people at work. In: Harrison R, Reeve F, Hanson A *et al*, editors. *Supporting Lifelong Learning. Vol 1: Perspectives on Learning*. London: Open University with Routledge/Falmer, 2002.

9 Bowler I. The skills escalator in primary care: developing new roles for the primary healthcare team. *Work Based Learning in Primary Care*. 2003; **1**: 12–18.

10 Boud D, Solomon N. Repositioning universities and work. In: Boud D, Solomon N, editors. *Work-based Learning. A new higher education*. Buckingham: SRHE and OUP, 2001.

11 Staley M. Evaluating an in-house education programme. *Work Based Learning in Primary Care*. 2003; **1**: 69–74.

12 NHS 24. accessed at: www.nhs24.com.

13 Cole M. Reflection in healthcare practice: why is it useful and how might it be done? *Work Based Learning in Primary Care*. 2005; **3**: 13–22.

14 Jackson N. Assessment and work based learning in primary care. *Work Based Learning in Primary Care*. 2003; **1**: 89–92.

15 National Institute for Clinical Excellence *Chronic Heart Failure. Management of chronic heart failure in adults in primary and secondary care. Clinical guideline 5*. London: National Institute for Clinical Excellence, 2003.

16 Cole M. Capture and measurement of work-based and informal learning: a discussion of the issues in regard to contemporary health care practice. *Work Based Learning in Primary Care*. 2004; **2**: 118–25.

17 Sandars J. Work based learning: a social network perspective. *Work Based Learning in Primary Care*. 2005; **3**: 4–12.

18 Burton J. Self-assessment, peer assessment and third party assessment: significance for work based learning. *Work Based Learning in Primary Care* 2004; **3**: 1–3.

19 Jackson N, Burton J. Work based learning in primary care: where to next? In: Burton J, Jackson N, editors. *Work Based Learning in Primary Care*. Abingdon: Radcliffe Medical Press, 2003.

20 Eraut M. Factors affecting learning in the workplace. Paper presented at the Work Based Learning in Primary Care conference, reported in Fowler I. 2004.Vol 1: 3.

21 Burton J, Perkins J. Accounts of personal learning in primary care. *Work Based Learning in Primary Care*. 2003; **1**: 19–32.

22 McKee A, Watts M. Practice and Professional Development Plans in East Anglia: a case of politics, policy and practice. *Work Based Learning in Primary Care*. 2003. **1**: I.

23 Dewey J. *Democracy and Education*. New York, Free Press, 1916.

24 Stenhouse L. *An Introduction to Curriculum Research and Development*. London: Heinemann, 1975.

25 McKee A. *Competence Based Assessment in Higher Education: the case of the standards methodology*. Centre for Applied Research in Education, at the British Educational Research Association, 1995.

26 Launer J, Burton J. Why do education and training fail to prepare us for the job in hand? *Work Based Learning in Primary Care*. 2004; **2**: 109–10.

27 *The Book of Common Prayer*. Second Collect. For Peace. Oxford: Oxford University Press, 1963.

28 Department of Health. *A First Class Service: quality in the new NHS*. London: Department of Health, 1998.

Chapter 6

E-learning: it's learning, Jim, but not as we know it!

Alan Gillies

The title to this chapter is a misappropriation of an immortal line from the original Star Trek television series where Dr McCoy says to Captain James T Kirk, ' It's life, Jim, but not as we know it!'

What is e-learning?

E-learning is becoming an important part of life in general and the NHS in particular. Every NHS trust should have an e-learning strategy. Why?

Because it's a good thing, apparently. The late great Douglas Adams, himself a great fan of technology and information technology specifically, once wrote the line 'Bypasses? You have to build bypasses'. Perhaps e-learning applications are the new bypasses for the NHS. In Douglas Adams' book, his main character couldn't understand what was so great about place B that people from place A had to rush past place C on a bypass to get there.

There will be many people uncomfortable with technology who like learning things by reading books, going on courses, or going to ask their friendly NHS librarian for the information they need who will feel that e-learning is an unnecessary and unwelcome intrusion.

However, viewed sensibly, and in my experience evangelists and Luddites rarely view anything sensibly, e-learning can provide useful tools and facilities to help people learn.

Let's start with a definition. There are many. Here's one I like:

> E-learning is the effective learning process created by combining digitally delivered content with (learning) support and services.
>
> Open and Distance Learning Council

I like it because it emphasises learning and recognises the need for support and services. Also it's not too long, and not as extreme as the comment from a friend and colleague:

> There's no such thing as e-learning, there's only learning, which occurs in the brains of people.

Whilst unhelpful in defining e-learning, this is a note of good caution we should remember when getting carried away with clever technology. To explore the nature of e-learning further here are my 10 myths and commandments about e-learning.

The 10 myths and commandments about e-learning

Let me start with five myths I have heard about e-learning.

Box 6.1 The myths of e-learning

1 **E-learning is always best.**
No, it's not best! Sorry, but sometimes it's just not appropriate!

2 **E-learning means that staff don't need time away from work to learn.**
Just because e-learning can be flexible, doesn't mean that staff don't need time to learn. Too often, it's a way of pushing learning from work time into home time.

3 **Rich media (that's fancy video to you and me!) produces better learning.**
Used appropriately, video technology can be very effective but it's only a tool. It can be used badly or inappropriately like any tool.

4 **Putting books, lecture notes or even videos of lectures onto the internet or CD is e-learning.**
Lectures are often a very poor way of communicating a bland body of knowledge. By taking away the physical presence of the lecturer we actually reduce the effectiveness of the delivery further. There is no guarantee that any actual learning will ensue.

5 **E-learning is passive not active.**
Because many of the early attempts at e-learning are in reality not much more than putting existing material onto the web or a CD as a distribution medium, this myth has grown up. It should not have to be like that.

And now here are my commandments.

Box 6.2 The commandments of e-learning

1 **E-learning should be 11% E and 88% learning.**
This is factually correct. There are eight times as many letters in 'learning' as in 'E'. However, more importantly, it is metaphorically correct. It is important for the design of e-learning to focus upon the learning, and what you wish to achieve from a learning perspective. Only then can you decide which technology you wish to use from chalk to streamed video.

2 **Learning should involve multiple techniques.**
Learners have different styles, and you will need different methods to deal effectively with this. Good teachers do this all the time intuitively. Different problems require different approaches, and you will need to use different methods here too. Within your multiple approaches, you may use e- and non-e- approaches. This is called blended learning.

---

3 **The e-learning experience should be better than alternative learning experiences.**
    If not, why use it?
4 **E-learning will succeed if you engage the learner in a two way process.**
    Effective learning requires the learner to actively participate. E-learning needs to move beyond the transmission of knowledge to engage the user. There are many ways to do this which we shall explore later in this chapter.
5 **E-learning should use a variety of media and transmission methods, as determined by the needs of the application.**
    Some writers have argued that 'true' e-learning is associated with a particular medium or mode of delivery. Once again, technology is being put at the centre. Determine the needs of your application and your intended audience and then use appropriate technology to deliver your learning.

Types of e-learning

In reality, and in spite of the efforts of fans or salesmen of particular technologies, e-learning is extremely diverse. We shall seek to classify the types of e-learning according to a range of criteria.

E-learning applications can be classified according to any number of criteria. We shall focus upon the following two criteria, for the pragmatic reason that I think they can tell us the most about an e-learning application:

* purpose of learning
* delivery mechanism and environment.

Purpose of learning

One of the key characteristics of e-learning is to think about its purpose. E-learning has often become associated with 'just in time' learning to meet the requirements of professional development or mandatory training, e.g. replacement of the annual fire lecture. It is also increasingly being used as a replacement for face-to-face teaching in higher and further education to enable students to achieve qualifications without having to attend classroom sessions, e.g. Masters in Health Informatics at the University of Central Lancashire or the University of Bath. In reality, these characterise two ends of a spectrum.

To consider e-learning in these contexts, here are my thoughts as to the benefits and drawbacks of using e-learning for these purposes, shown in Table 6.1. I have added a face symbol to suggest whether a perceived benefit is realised in practice. Where a claimed benefit appears difficult to realise in practice, I have put a frown, and where a claimed disadvantage may be overcome with good design, I have added a smile.

Table 6.1 Benefits and drawbacks of using e-learning

Purpose	Strengths of e-learning	Weaknesses of e-learning	Opportunities from e-learning	Threats to e-learning
Just in time learning	Flexibility of time of delivery Flexibility of place of delivery Efficiency of delivery	Reduced opportunity for instant feedback ☺ Increased passivity of learner ☺	Link to training needs analysis tools	Risk of incoherent learning Time not available
Formal qualifications	Flexibility of time of delivery Flexibility of place of delivery Efficiency of delivery ☹	Reduced opportunity for instant feedback ☺ Increased passivity of learner ☺	Bigger market for providers Integration and automation of management functions ☹ Opportunity to establish a learning community ☹ Basis for a variety of blended routes	Competition Time not available

Delivery mechanism and environment

Whilst technology should not overshadow what we are trying to do from a learning perspective, it may constrain what we can do. However, remember that we can combine methods to achieve an optimum solution. For example, internet-based communications can be used to supplement a CD-ROM-based solution. E-learning is generally delivered through one of three methods.

1 Read-only disk, e.g. CD-ROM.
2 Open distributed, e.g. internet.
3 Closed distributed, e.g. Virtual Learning Environment.

Currently, within the health sector there are examples of e-learning applications for a variety of purposes using a variety of delivery mechanisms. If you have been involved with e-learning, how did you find your experience? Do you recognise the SWOT analyses in Table 6.2?

Should you be using e-learning?

Some of you will be potential providers of e-learning, many of you will be potential users of e-learning. Should you be using e-learning at all? Many of us in

Table 6.2 Analysis of e-learning delivery mechanisms

Purpose	Strengths	Weaknesses	Opportunities	Threats
Read-only disk, e.g. CD-ROM	Version control Cost Universality	Adaptability Failure to support communication	Low cost of duplication	Out of date material
Open distributed, e.g. internet	Widespread access to internet	Dependence upon external links Connection speed	Growth of broadband access Opportunity to establish a learning community ☹	Internet security threats, e.g. viruses Version control
Closed distributed, e.g. Virtual Learning Environment	Widespread access via the internet Controlled access	Dependence upon external links Connection speed Closed nature of systems Cost of setup Complexity Inflexibility	Integration and automation of management functions ☹ Opportunity to establish a learning community	Proprietary nature of systems, internet security threats, e.g. viruses Version control ☺

reality have little choice. Even providers may be under pressure from managers or external agencies to embrace the new technology. However, in case you have a choice or just want reassurance that it's worth using the technology, here's my checklist of good reasons to use e-learning. You don't need all of them to make it worthwhile, but you need more than one so, for example, accessibility is often a plus, but not enough on its own!

Box 6.3 Alan's good reasons for using e-learning

1 It increases accessibility to learning.
2 It enables new and interesting ways of learning.
3 It provides direct access to a wide range of primary sources.
4 It facilitates the formation of a community from a geographically diverse group of learners.
5 It targets learning to training needs and prevents repetition of unnecessary learning.
6 It allows the material to be kept up to date.
7 It allows for the development of locally relevant materials in support of core generic materials.

> 8   It allows you to provide a collective learning experience, e.g. based around an electronic scenario to a distributed group of learners.
> 9   It provides a common learning experience across a wide and distributed group of students.
> 10 It facilitates inclusion of learners for students who would not have access to learning in other ways.

If you have been involved with e-learning before, how many did you score?

0: Life can only get better!
1–3: It seems unlikely that e-learning was a good choice!
4–6: This was e-learning that is better than average!
7–9: If you were provider, well done, if a learner, you were very lucky!
10: Wow!

Active e-learning

The secret of good comedy is . . . timing! The secret of effective learning is active learning:

In the good old days, before e-learning was widely thought of, I was a lecturer at a university in North West England. One of the graduates from the course I taught on went to work for a friend of mine immediately after university.

With the graduate unaware of the connection, my friend asked him if he had been lectured by a Dr Gillies. 'Oh yes!' was the reply and for the next 10 minutes he recounted what I had talked about in the lectures at great length and also what was wrong with it.

When he had finished, my friend asked what his impressions of the other lecturers were. 'I don't remember them!' he said.

Engagement with learners may be achieved in a wide variety of ways, but it is essential that it is achieved by one means or another. Techniques designed to ensure that learning is active rather than passive may be individual or ideally collective, although this is not always possible.

Techniques to encourage active learning by individual learners may include the following:

• Questions for reflection or, in the case of formal qualifications, assignments that require the learner to apply the knowledge gained to their own situation.
• Multiple choice questions.

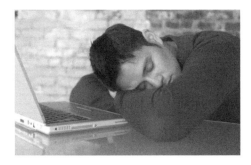 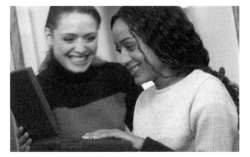

- Scenarios with questions to consider.
- Use of narrative with characters with whom the learners may identify.

Techniques to encourage collective active learning may include the following.

- Questions to start electronic group discussions.
- Scenarios to discuss electronically in real time or over a designated period.
- Establishment of an electronic community to enable knowledge sharing beyond the bounds of any specific e-learning.

It's all in the blend

Actually there's a real debate on that one between the drinkers of blended whiskies and the single malts. The title of this section was used by a major whisky company to promote their blended whisky, but it could equally have been written as a truism about e-learning.

One day a few years ago, I first read the term 'blended learning'. I thought what a good idea it was, until I realised that blended learning was in reality what I and most educators had been using for years. Blended learning is the use of a variety of techniques to promote effective learning. Usually these days it specifically refers to the use of e-learning techniques alongside the use of conventional materials. It refers to a continuous spectrum with all electronic learning at one end and all non-electronic learning at the other.

To illustrate the point, consider our own postgraduate health informatics courses (sorry to be parochial, but it's what I know best!). They run in two modes, which we tend to refer to as 'distance' and 'local' delivery. Both are based upon a range of core electronic materials provided on CD-ROM and via a dedicated online learning environment. In both cases, discussion is offered by

Table 6.3 Different blends

Group	Advantages	Disadvantages
'Distance'	Low attendance requirement facilitates involvement by students from Vancouver to Kent	Less direct contact
		Greater dependence upon technology
	Greater diversity of student population	Some students worry about lack of face-to-face contact
	Residential highly regarded by students: more informal than workshops	
'Local'	Strong group identity	Regular attendance required at local workshops
	Good local employer support	Less variety in peer group
	Reassurance for students worried about dependence upon technology	

an electronic forum and support by email, telephone or the option of coming into the University for a face-to-face meeting.

The significance different is that whilst both groups get a component delivered as face-to-face sessions, one is in the form of regular local workshops, the other in a single weekend residential per semester. This provides a different blend for each group with different features (*see* Table 6.3).

E-learning is rarely able to match the best human-led learning in terms of the ability to respond to individual learning styles, or the needs of a wide variety of problems.

However, a rich blend of multiple learning methods can enable the best of each method to be exploited. In the real world, the advantages of blended learning are often sacrificed on the grounds of cost or geographical location.

Standards for e-learning

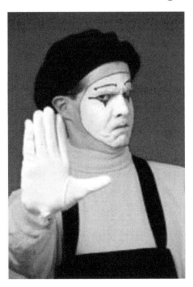

Standards are not intrinsically interesting. I know this. However, this bit is important so please not skip it and I shall try to make it as short as possible and maybe even a bit interesting.

To help, you can skip most of it, unless you plan to develop or buy your own e-learning. Coco will be back to tell you when you can skip to the next bit!

Standards are important for a number of reasons.

- Standards mean that electronic resources developed elsewhere will run on your computer. There are standards about your PC, CDs, DVDs, the internet, the pages themselves. In an ideal world, they work. When they work, you can ignore them. They're like the engine under the bonnet of your car: most of us don't want to know how it works, we just want it to carry on working!
- Standards are particularly important for including people with specific needs. Your Internet Explorer browser is very tolerant of inconsistencies in web pages and other code. An audio reader to allow a blind person to access the same page of material is unable to be that flexible. This is no longer just an aspiration. Recent legislation requires all providers to take all reasonable steps to ensure equality of access.
- Specific standards for e-learning materials have been developed to allow learning objects from one e-learning programme to work in another. Some authors claim this is essential for the future. Some of us are less convinced.

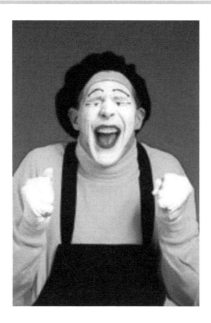

Ok, if you never want to develop or buy materials yourself, you can skip to the next section heading.

But it's not been so bad so far, and I promise I'll keep it brief. After all the Editor only gave me one chapter to cover all of e-learning, and I haven't got to the pictures yet!

And whether you skip the next bit or not, remember, accessible materials are required by law!

The first level of standards that e-learning should comply with are accessibility standards. The first essential is that the HTML code in which web-based materials will be written conforms to standards defined by the World Wide Web consortium. They additionally provide design guidance to ensure accessibility for as many users as possible. For more information go to www.w3.org.

The next step up in standards is to build your e-learning in discrete learning objects that are SCORM compliant. This is designed to enable you to take a learning object from one application and use it in another, and many NHS organisations will insist on SCORM-compliant applications.

There are a number of problems that limit my enthusiasm for SCORM compliance.

- It is overkill for many applications.
- It requires expensive editing software to produce the applications.
- The learning objects themselves are not so readily transferred to other delivery modes, whereas an HTML-based application can be transferred from online environments to CDs and back again.

SCORM compliance is useful in certain environments, for example in a big dedicated e-learning system where the metadata specified within SCORM can be used to track users through the system. If you need the sophistication that it offers, then you need to read several books larger than this, so I'll stop there!

Beyond substitution

Hopefully, by now, you have an appreciation of some of the key principles of e-learning; you will also have gathered that I do not believe that e-learning is a panacea. It is a well-established truism in other applications of information technology that benefits accrue not from the technology itself, but from changes in working practices that are facilitated by the use of the new technology.

A number of models have been developed to help understand how technology impacts upon organisations and how they become more 'mature' in their use of the technology. We shall consider the impact of e-learning upon organisations in terms of five phases:

1 *ad hoc*
2 substitution
3 strategic
4 innovative
5 embedded.

Ad hoc

At first, technology is adopted by enthusiasts or early adopters, as they have come to be known. Implementation is limited, and tends to be based in pilots or experiments. Thus, an organisation may introduce a few e-learning courses to see how the staff react. In reality, limited benefits will accrue; however, it may enthuse some of the early adopters to become local champions and to drive developments forward.

Substitution

In the next phase, e-learning is more widely adopted and usage focuses upon substitution of existing provision. Thus, in a 'just in time' learning situation, the annual fire lecture may be substituted by an online course. In a more formal educational context, lectures are substituted by materials designed to convey the lecture material in a didactic fashion, either text based or by video presentations of lectures, tutorials replaced by threaded or real-time discussion groups conducted online.

Strategic

To progress beyond the substitution of specific learning interventions, the organisation must start to think strategically. The strategic view should consider amongst other things:

- organisational goals for embracing e-learning
- characteristics and instances of learning applications that require or suit e-learning
- characteristics and instances of learning applications that are not well suited to e-learning
- organisational technological capacity for embracing e-learning
- organisational human capacity for embracing e-learning
- timescales for meeting goals.

An organisation at this stage of development is characterised by having a coherent approach to e-learning across the organisation. A major challenge is to retain the innovation and enthusiasm of the e-learning champions within a systemic framework

Innovative

Only when organisations start to move beyond the constraints of traditional learning will maximum benefits accrue. This happens when the organisation starts to use technology to do things that it simply could not do without the technology, rather than simply replacing the existing *modus operandi*. The most dramatic examples from history are the Industrial Revolution, which produced massive efficiency gains not just from using new technology but organising the work in new much more efficient ways. Arguably, a similar thing happened when computers became networked, leading to the internet and its associated applications, email and the World Wide Web.

E-learning can lead to a range of innovations which can make a big improvement either in learning or the management of learning, including:

- Integration and automation of administration processes
- Linking to training needs analysis tools
- New ways of learning
- Establishment of virtual communities who may be geographically disparate but linked by a common subject interest
- Instant access to primary sources.

Embedded

At its most effective, e-learning becomes an embedded part of the organisation. It is highly likely that at this point, the organisation ceases to think in terms of e-learning at all, but rather simply uses technology as part of its learning processes. E-learning is simply another approach to learning and its use is determined by pragmatic assessment of the best learning methods available.

Examples of e-learning

To finish this chapter, we will illustrate the points made by referring to a number of examples of e-learning applications and highlighting some of the more novel features of each application. I have restricted my examples to my own applications for copyright reasons.

Case study I: Clinical governance material

This application was developed for Radcliffe Publishing Limited, and is designed for a healthcare audience. It seeks to provide an introduction to clinical governance in an interesting way and with a light touch.

Some of its key features are:
- A need for timeliness in response to a changing policy agenda
- Assessment with instant feedback
- Separation of online links into a library of resources to permit CD distribution and easy maintenance

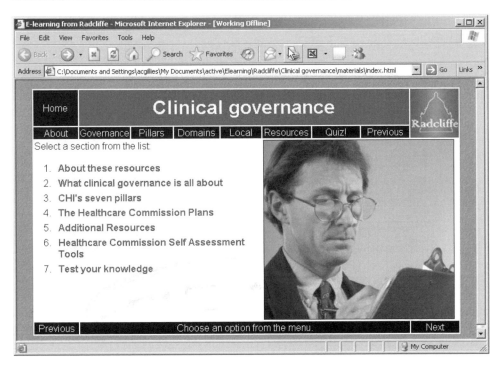

Figure 6.1 Clinical governance e-learning application for Radcliffe Publishing

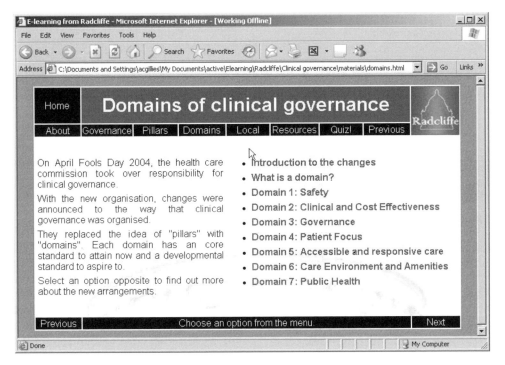

Figure 6.2 Adaptation to meet the needs of the Healthcare Commission

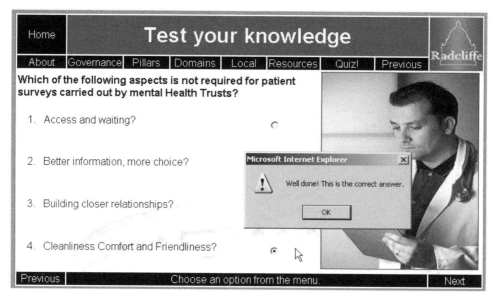

Figure 6.3 Question with positive response

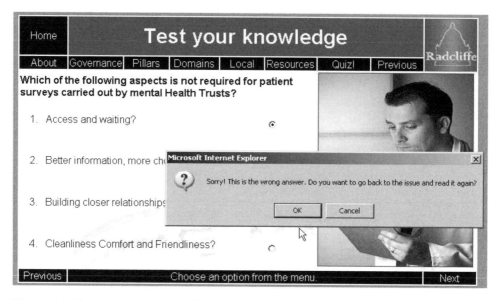

Figure 6.4 The wrong answer leads to a feedback response

Clinical governance policy changes rapidly. There is a need for timeliness and e-learning can be updated more easily than a book, e.g. on the establishment of the Healthcare Commission (*see* Figure 6.2).

Multiple choice questions were used to provide instant feedback. If a correct answer is shown the learner receives a positive response (*see* Figure 6.3).

However, if the wrong answer is given, the technology adds value by offering the learner the chance to return to the relevant section of learning (*see* Figure 6.4).

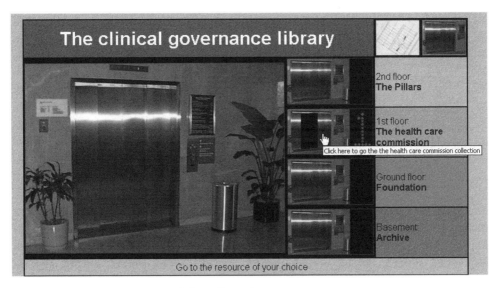

Figure 6.5 The entrance hall of the collected resources

Finally, to facilitate CD-ROM distribution and maintenance, the external links to resources are collated into an online library (*see* Figure 6.5).

Case study 2: The MSc in Health informatics

Since 2000, the MSc in Health Informatics at the University of Central Lancashire has run in a largely electronic blended mode. Initially offered in CD plus internet mode, it is now offered additionally via the University's virtual learning environment to provide more facilities to staff and students.

Features of the materials are:

- Strong visual metaphors for the virtual campus and library
- wide use of primary sources
- use of reflective activities to promote active learning.

The visual metaphor is emphasised through the use of 'floors' for different purposes, linked by a lift (*see* Figures 6.6–6.9)

The course makes wide use of primary sources collected in the virtual library, available to all at www.healthlibrary.org.uk, and reflective activities to promote active learning (*see* Figure 6.10).

Case study 3: E-learning for patients and the public

The third case study is an application commissioned by ADITUS, the North West NHS Library Service, who wanted an application to help patients find and critique health information.

A different style was adopted in view of the target audience, with the application following Joe as he sought the information he required, allowing the learner to visit the same resources as Joe, mirroring the character's experience for the learner.

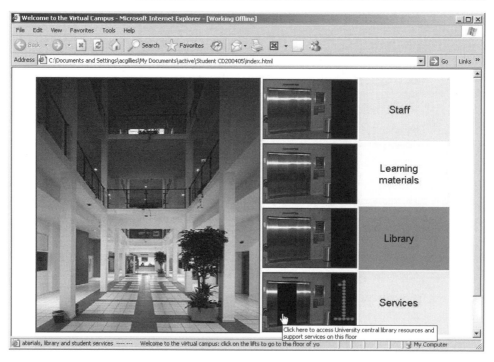

Figure 6.6 Entrance hall with lift at floor 1

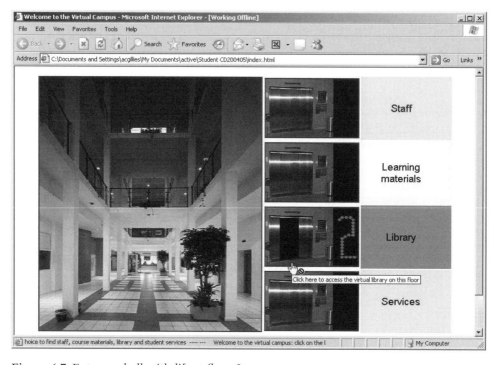

Figure 6.7 Entrance hall with lift at floor 2

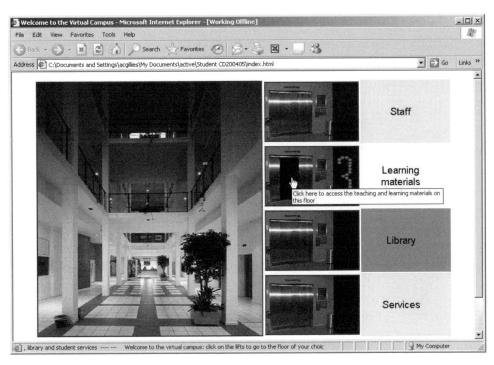

Figure 6.8 Entrance hall with lift at floor 3

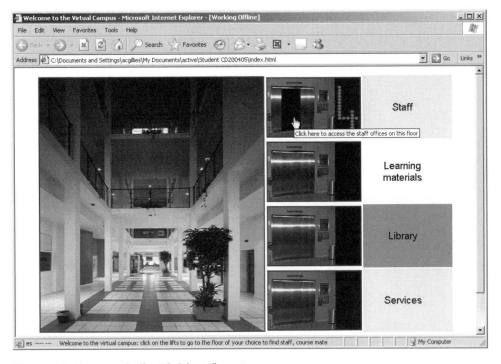

Figure 6.9 Entrance hall with lift at floor 4

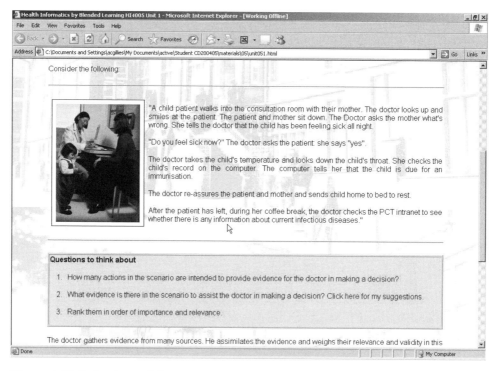

Figure 6.10 Reflective activity

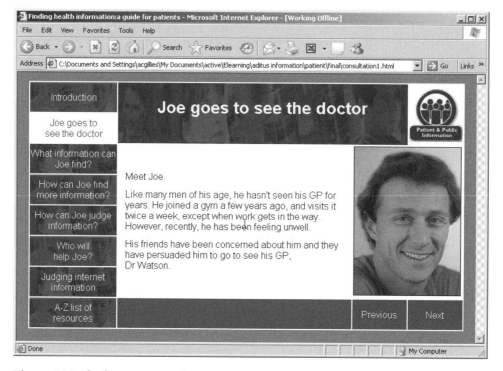

Figure 6.11 The learner meets Joe

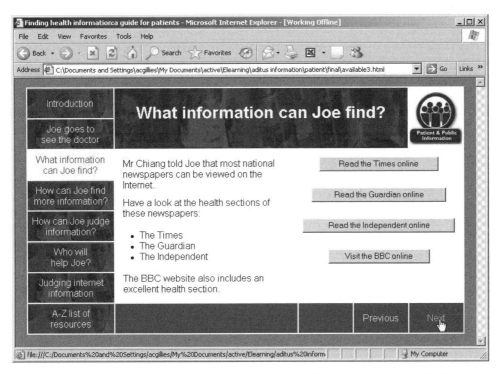

Figure 6.12 The learner goes to the library with Joe and reads the papers with him

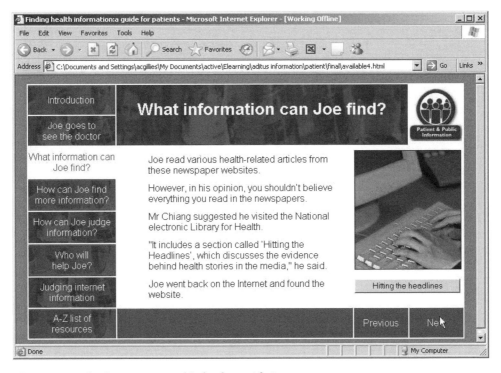

Figure 6.13 The learner goes a bit further with Joe

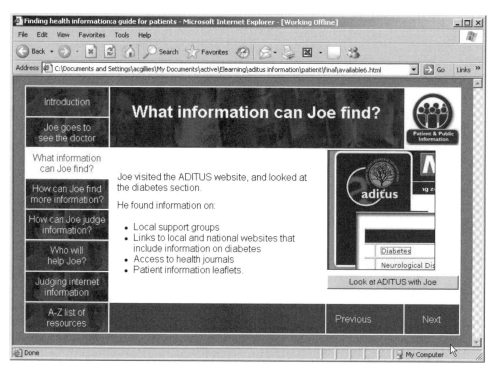

Figure 6.14 The learner explores websites with Joe

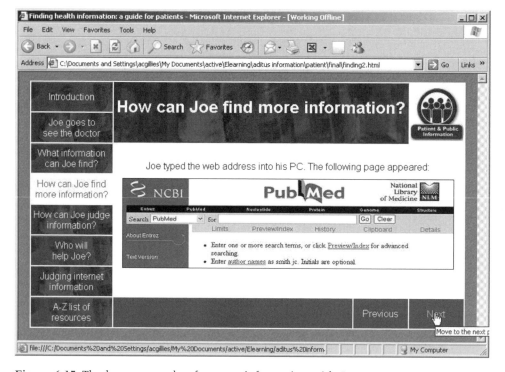

Figure 6.15 The learner searches for more information with Joe

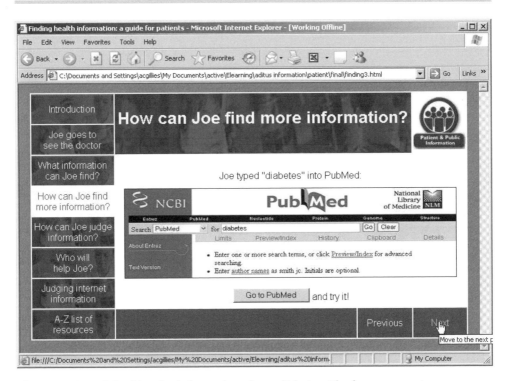

Figure 6.16 Joe's looking for information about diabetes. The learner can, too

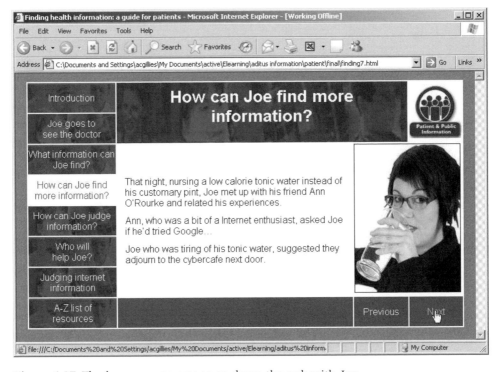

Figure 6.17 The learner even gets to go down the pub with Joe

The case studies seek to show how a variety of techniques can be used to address a range of applications.

Bibliography

Ideally, this should be a list of online resources. Unfortunately, sites have a habit of changing. Still, the following should hopefully be still there when you read this:

- www.aditus.nhs.uk where you should be able to find the patient resource in case study 3
- www.alangillies.com: my site, with samples of e-learning applications
- www.healthlibrary.org.uk the virtual library developed for our students
- www.nhsu.nhs.uk where much of the NHS effort is concentrated
- www.w3.org OK, one for the anoraks, but it's the definitive source of information about the web.

However, as this should be an 'active' learning experience, why not email me with your comments and questions at professor@alangillies.com? If we get enough interest we could set up a discussion group for the whole book!

Chapter 7

Appraisal for Allied Health Professions

Wendy M White

Background

Appraisal has long been considered to be essential in managing effective organ-isations. The NHS has an interesting history in engaging people in accepting and systematically deploying appraisal. Prior to the government's modernisation agenda which has led to a mandatory requirement for all trusts to have an appraisal process in place, the most systematic previous effort at supporting appraisal implementation was the NHS Individual Performance Review (IPR) scheme, introduced in 1986.

Since then a number of national drivers have established appraisal as essential. *The New NHS: modern, dependable*[1] confirms that:

> Health professionals, professional bodies and local employers need to discuss a locally based approach to CPD, centred on the service needs of the community and the learning needs of the individual.

The document *Working Together: securing a quality workforce for the NHS*[2] has as one of its strategic aims to:

> Ensure that the NHS has a quality workforce, in the right numbers, with the right skills, and diversity, organised in the right way to deliver the Government's service objectives for health and social care.

Having in place a training and development plan for the majority of healthcare professionals is a key target from this.

A First Class Service[1] identifies the importance of 'investing in lifelong learning' and the need for this to be supported by practical issues including 'the role of monitoring, peer review and appraisal'.

Many professional groups have made the link between regular appraisal and the professional revalidation process.

Currently the Department of Health identifies the primary aim of NHS appraisal as being to identify personal and professional development needs.

In addition, appraisal has currency thanks to the explicit links being established between the process and improvements to the quality of care to patients. Recent research by Borrill and West[3] concluded that HR accounts for 33% of hospital variance in patient mortality. The three contributory factors include appraisal, training and staff working in teams, the strongest link being appraisal.

Overall, the National Staff Survey indicates that 66% of staff across the service now receive appraisal. However, the challenge facing HR professionals, line managers and individual practitioners is to improve the effectiveness of the appraisal experience. The current survey indicates that the effectiveness can be variable (35%).

It is likely that most organisations, professional groups and individual staff members subscribe to the benefits that appraisal can bring to patients and staff. The biggest challenge is to ensure that a sustainable, flexible, reliable and effective system for appraisal is systematically deployed throughout the organisation and across all staff groups.

In this chapter appraisal is considered in general: its benefits, some of the related issues to successful deployment of appraisal, the impact of *Agenda for Change* (*AfC*) and in particular how team appraisal has been successfully implemented.

What is appraisal?

The answer to this question according to the *IPR Training Knowledge Book*[4] is:

> . . . essentially a process of agreeing job objectives and targets, then monitoring and evaluating their subsequent achievement.

This 'process' can be questionnaire-focused, use rating scales, be results-oriented, competency-based, seek views from multi-levels and multi-sources, for example 360° feedback (*see* Chapter 8). A key component of any approach is a degree of self-appraisal. The appraisal interview is the opportunity to share, reflect and look forward using any of these processes.

An effective appraisal can help to:

- clarify role expectations
- assess current performance
- acknowledge and appreciate staff contributions
- identify areas of improvement
- help staff to fulfil their potential
- set targets or objectives
- support the organisation in succession planning
- improve working relationships.

This can benefit both the individual and the organisation by:

- improving individual and organisational performance through the cascade of organisational and personal objectives
- identifying individual and corporate training and development needs
- systematically planning career and professional development
- aiding succession planning
- improving morale
- demonstrating the value the organisation places on its staff.

So, who needs to be appraised? The answer is everyone.[5] Why? Because the benefits are pervasive for the organisation, the department, the individual and ultimately the patient.[3]

The benefits of appraisal

The benefits for the organisation from appraisal include:

- acting as a key component in changing culture
- promoting more open styles of management and leadership
- influencing collective values
- devolving authority, accountability and responsibility to the appropriate levels
- creating opportunities for organisational learning
- seeking better value for money through targeted staff development that ensures both the capacity and capability to deliver business objectives.

The benefits for the department are the:

- identification of common/team goals and improved team working
- clarification of authority, accountability and responsibility
- aiding of succession planning
- opportunity to draw on ideas from all staff
- improved communications.

The benefits for the individual are to:

- receive positive encouragement and recognition of achievement
- have the opportunity to give feedback
- formally review and take stock of past performance
- identify career pathways and immediate development needs and contribute to continuing professional development
- clarify expectations for the coming year.

The appraisal process

Appraisal is most effective when it forms part of a performance management process. This means linking the performance of the individual employees to the achievements, outputs and targets of the organisation overall.

Organisational performance is dependent upon the performance of those working for it. Increased motivation, a sense of making a difference along with goal achievement can enhance staff morale. Making this link through the appraisal process is essential to individual and organisational success.

Whatever type of appraisal is used it is essential that there are clear objectives for everyone which are aligned with the organisation's strategic goals and a clear personal development plan.

Clarifying who the appraiser is must be an essential first step. In most instances the person undertaking the appraisal is the manager or supervisor of the individual being appraised. However, for supervised placements, in matrix management situations (for example where a specialty has day-to-day supervision but professional accountability elsewhere) or joint management arrangements (for example where the service is provided in an acute setting but managed from within primary care) the responsibility may be less clear. Practical arrangements about seeking information from people knowledgeable about an individual's performance are important for whoever conducts the appraisal interview.

There are three key steps in the appraisal process:

1 preparation
2 the appraisal meeting
3 the follow-up.

Preparation

Preparation is an essential part of appraisal and starts with the vital process of self-appraisal. The appraiser needs to agree with the appraisee what form preparation will take and provide adequate time so that the preparation is both realistic and meaningful.

To support this preparation the appraiser needs, at least seven days before the appraisal, to:

- answer any questions the appraisee may have about the purpose or outcomes of appraisal
- provide details of any plans and departmental objectives for the coming year
- provide any other information which either party feels would be helpful, e.g. the appraiser's current work objectives or those of the manager above the appraiser
- agree, if necessary, if there is any third party the appraiser needs to seek performance information from
- agree how self-appraisal of past and current performance would be best undertaken.

This last point is very important. Self-appraisal of performance is key to ensuring joint participation in the process and establishing good two-way communication.

Self-appraisal

Options for self-appraisal include:

1 A structured self assessment form

> **Box 7.1 Self-assessment form**
>
> **Self-appraisal**
> Using a limited number of focused questions will effectively get both the manager and member of staff to think about performance. An indicative list below covers often used questions.
>
> **The job**
> - What is the overall purpose of your job – what does it exist to do?
> - In what way could your job be improved?
> - Has your job changed significantly in the past 12 months? If so, how?
> - In what way could you improve the job you do?
> - What is it about your present job you like/dislike?
> - What changes in your job would you like to make?
> - In your present job, what extra skills or knowledge would you find helpful?
> - How do you work most effectively?
> - What are your key skills?
>
> **Achievement**
> - What were your major achievements last year in relation to your agreed objectives?
> - What do you think has brought about your achievements?
> - What important abilities do you have that are not being used?

Improvement/problem solving
- What were your major disappointments last year in relation to your agreed objectives?
- How would you like to see your working relationships develop/change?
- Which areas of your work have proved demanding/frustrating/difficult/disappointing?

Box 7.2 Work areas

Career
- Do you have skills/knowledge developed elsewhere, which are not used in your job?
- What do you wish to be doing over the next five years?

Education, training and development
- What personal development needs do you have?
- In what ways do you feel you could meet your personnel development needs?
- In what aspects of your job do you feel you need more experience or training?
- To help your personal development, what additional things might be done by: your manager, yourself, the trust.
- What skills/knowledge/competency need to be developed to help you do your job?

Objectives
- What do you consider to be your objectives over the next 12 months?
- What key tasks have you been involved in over the past year?
- What did you find easy/difficult to do? Why?
- What are the objectives of your department section for the coming year?
- What is or could be your contribution to these objectives?

2   An agreement to customise a set of standard questions as shown in Box 7.2.

A less structured approach could focus on a number of general and/or specific questions:

- In what way could you improve the job you do?
- How do you work most effectively?
- Which areas of your work have proved demanding/frustrating/difficult/disappointing?
- What do you consider to be your objectives over the next 12 months?

Agreement about sharing the self-appraisal information can be negotiated between the appraiser and appraisee. Some people like to use their self-assessment as a personal *aide memoire* for the meeting, others are happy to share the information a few days before the meeting to allow both parties to prepare fully.

The practical preparation for the interview to take place has to be planned: time, place, without interruptions, etc. as well as reviewing key information from:

- other key contributors on performance
- self-appraisal information (if being shared)
- review of organisational objectives
- review of departmental objectives
- review of personal objectives
- reflection on last year's objectives and personal development plan.

The appraisal meeting

Successful appraisal discussions rely on good preparation and open, honest, mutual, two-way communication. Confidentiality is essential. Sufficient time must be given and there must be no interruptions.

There is differing opinion on how formal/informal an appraisal meeting should be and obviously reviewers' styles are likely to differ significantly. Of greater importance is that the meeting is well structured and the nature of appraisal and development review is advantageous. A likely structure would be:

1 appraiser confirms purpose of meeting and desired outcomes
2 appraiser outlines the structure of meeting, confirms what will be recorded and agrees process with appraisee.

Joint 'looking back'

1 Appraisee input on self-assessment of performance and past objectives.
2 Feedback from appraiser and exchange of views.
3 Review of personal development plan.
4 Make notes of what needs continuing/further action.

Discuss the present

1 Departmental objectives.
2 Ideas for change/improvement in individual, team, organisational and service performance.
3 Make notes of any impact the discussion has on work objectives and PDP.

Look forward

1 Agree future action plans and objectives.
2 Review any outstanding personal development needs.
3 Fix appraisal review dates.
4 Agree when any 'deferred' items will be resolved.

It may be helpful, however, to reflect on a few 'dos and don'ts' (*see* Table 7.1).

Identifying, setting and agreeing objectives

Agreeing individual objectives, aligned with those of the trust, is a key purpose of appraisal. Objectives can be divided into three different types.

1 **Continuing standard of performance:** Applies to objectives where the standard agreed simply defines a level of performance to continue getting the results we want to maintain.

2 **Performance improvement:** Applies to objectives where the standard agreed raises the level of performance to improve our results.

3 **Project:** Applies to objectives that are one-off events and most often involve a task needing to be completed to a certain standard within a specific time frame.

To be effective, all objectives need to be SMART (*see* Table 7.2).

Table 7.1 Dos and don'ts of appraisal

Do:	Don't:
Agree the agenda and time frame – then respect it	Disengage from the process
	Forget to use your preparation material
Actively listen	Agree to objectives that are unrealistic
Be prepared for feedback and make it constructive	But accept that you need evidence why they are
Use conversation that is evidence based	Dwell on feedback that you perceive as unfair or negative – state your feelings and be prepared to move on
Focus on areas that need attention or on differences	
But if there are serious differences in one area, defer and move on	
Be clear and accurate about capacity for workload	
Respect the process by concentrating on performance not personality	
Give praise where due	
Be specific about successes and failures	

Table 7.2 'SMART' objectives

Specific	With regard to what is intended.
Measurable and monitored	Based on performance criteria that can be used to assess whether the objective is being achieved.
Agreed and activity based	With the people responsible for achievement.
	Clear about what activities are involved in achieving the objective.
Realistic and relevant	Capable of being achieved within the time and resources available. Relevant to the needs of the trust and the people involved.
Timed and timely	Set to a timetable that will give signposts for fulfilment and a date for completion.
	Set at the right time.

The follow-up

The nature of appraisal means that meeting is the start of a process as well as an end. The follow-up process will include the identified appraisal outcomes. These might be:

- Staff have agreed objectives for the forthcoming year, aligned to the organisation's strategic goals and business plan.
- A record of the appraisal detailing the objectives agreed by the appraiser and appraisee – each retaining a copy for future reference.

> Recording appraisal information could take up another chapter, and in practice many appraisal schemes are designed around the paperwork that staff are required to complete. Many failures of appraisal are due to an overemphasis on box-filling and ticking/grading assessment rather than listening to achievements and agreeing future developments.
>
> Forms used for appraisal range from single sheets to 'mini-dissertations'.

- Appropriate and agreed sharing of objective information to ensure congruence with organisational objectives, for example the appraising manager's manager (grandparent).
- A personal development plan that identifies their learning and development needs (shared as agreed for example with the Learning and Development team so that priorities for learning can be identified organisation-wide).

> **Box 7.3 Personal development plans (PDPs)**
>
> The production, monitoring and evaluation of PDPs as part of the appraisal process are important to:
>
> 1 identify the knowledge and skills individuals need to apply to their role
> 2 guide development that meets organisational and individual needs
> 3 promote equality and access to development interventions required to support development
> 4 help individuals learn and develop in their current role and gain job satisfaction for the future.
>
> An effective PDP sets clear goals and identifies the support, knowledge, skill or competence required to achieve agreed objectives, as well as identifying the support for professional or personal development.

Regular review dates ensure:

1 plans and key tasks are kept on track
2 standards are being achieved
3 opportunities to assess the effect of external factors
4 any necessary corrective action can be taken when it will be most effective.

Review need not be formal or time consuming and is ideally best integrated into day-to-day management activity. It could be planned to coincide with key milestones or before and after development activities. How often will depend on a range of things:

- The type of objectives agreed – their complexity and the type of tasks involved in meeting the objectives.
- The nature of an individual's work and their level of authority and accountability.
- The work environment particularly concerning numbers of staff and staff availability.
- An individual's knowledge, skills, experience and approach.
- The type of activities involved in the individual's development.

As a guide, an individual might expect to meet their reviewer for a routine review meeting two to three times a year.

Appraisal and Agenda for Change

The implementation of *Agenda for Change*[6] brings some important changes to appraisal by strengthening the focus on learning and development through the introduction of the NHS Knowledge and Skills Framework[7] (KSF) (*see* Box 7.4). NHS KSF provides the structure to support the development of individuals in their work in the post they currently hold, support individual career progression throughout an employee's working life and facilitates the development of services so that they better meet the needs of patients and the public.

The framework is made up of written generic descriptions of the knowledge and skills that individuals in the NHS need to apply in their post. The descriptions are referred to as 'dimensions'. There are 30 in total: six (the core dimensions) which apply to every post in the NHS, and 24 which are specific to different jobs. In order to use the framework, what is called a 'post outline' has been developed for every job. Post outlines focus on the job not an individual and consist of the six core dimensions and a number of the specific dimensions that have been identified as relevant to the post.

Box 7.4 KSF

The Knowledge and Skills Framework (KSF) is an important element of *Agenda for Change* – it recognises that post holders need learning and development to progress in their careers. Though the KSF is essentially a development tool it will also contribute to decisions about pay progression.

The knowledge and skills needed to do your job will be set out in a KSF outline.

- Your post will have a subset KSF outline – this represents the minimum knowledge and skills needed to do a job safely. When you meet this, you will progress through the Foundation Gateway.
- Your post will also have a full KSF outline – this represents the knowledge and skills needed at full development. You must meet this to progress through the Second Gateway.

KSF outlines are made up of 30 dimensions. These dimensions identify broad functions that are required by the NHS to enable it to provide a good-quality service to the public. Six core dimensions are relevant to everyone's job. They are:

1 Communication
2 Personal and people development
3 Health, safety and security
4 Service improvement
5 Quality
6 Equality and diversity.

The other 24 specific dimensions apply to some jobs but not others and are grouped in themes:

- Health & well-being (10)
- Estates & facilities (3)
- Information & knowledge (3)
- General (8).

Each dimension has four levels – your post will have a set level at which you will have to apply that particular dimension. Levels show advancing skill or knowledge requirements in the job.

You and your manager will agree a personal KSF profile showing how you compare with your job's KSF outline.

By examining the difference between your personal and the job KSF outline you and your manager will be able to identify and review your training needs as part of your development review. A personal development plan will then be agreed to enable you to continue to develop your skills further.

What is a development review?

A development review is an ongoing cycle of review, planning, development and evaluation for staff in the NHS linked to organisational and individual development needs. The development review is a partnership between an individual member of staff and their manager. The main purpose of the development review process is to:

- Review how individuals are applying knowledge and skills to meet the demands of their current post.
- Review the development needs of the individual member of staff.
- Identify the development that the individual needs over the next period of time.
- Plan how and when this development will take place and the date of the next review.

A personal development plan is agreed by an individual member of staff and their manager at the development review by mapping the staff member's present knowledge and skills against either a subset KSF outline – first post review – or a full KSF outline at subsequent reviews.

Source: *The KSF Handbook*

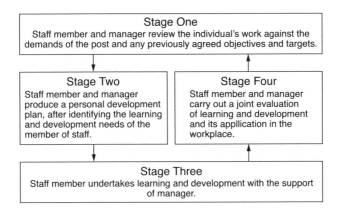

Figure 7.1 Stages of the KSF process

A post outline is an essential tool in every appraisal. Individual organisations have to make an early decision about the link between appraisal and the development review process heralded in *Agenda for Change*.

Local decisions are required to decide whether to keep the performance review process separate from the development review process or to include appraisal as part of the development review cycle. For all sorts of pragmatic reasons the latter is likely to happen in practice:

- time available to prepare for appraisals
- time required for development review
- time required to review evidence for pay progressions
- time to review performance for professional validation purposes
- time to support the subsequent development needs
- the need to link personal performance with departmental and corporate performance.

At the review the KSF outline is used to jointly match the current development level of the member of staff against the dimension demands of the post as detailed in the 'outline'. This will show the individual's current skills, knowledge and experience and identify any 'gaps' for development. From this a PDP is agreed which will identify the learning and development needs, set the objectives, detail how these will be met and agree what evidence is needed. Staff are supported in meeting the objectives of their PDP through a range of different learning opportunities and there will be regular PDP reviews to evaluate learning and how it has been applied to the individual's work. (Mandatory paperwork appears in the NHS Knowledge and Skills Framework and the Development Review Process.)[8]

Team appraisal

Traditional appraisal works on a one-to-one methodology where an identified supervisor typically reviews the performance and potential of an individual reporting to them. Perhaps more implicit is the emphasis and value that team working can play. Individual review can sometimes overlook the impact of the team contribution to an activity, objective, client care and treatment. Individual assessment of performance then has its limitations as progress may have been hindered or helped by a number of factors not routinely reviewed at an individual's appraisal.

The emphasis on effective team working would support the need to review team performance in a structured and systematic way that promotes the same kind of corporate, departmental, and individual benefit.

There are essentially two stages to team appraisal: first, a team event and second, meetings between individual team members and the team manager to agree personal development plans.

There is no one formula for the team event and they vary greatly according to a wide range of factors including size of team, nature of the team's work and working arrangements. It is unlikely, however, that it would be successful if team appraisal was included as part of another activity, such as a team meeting.

As in one-to-one appraisal, individual team members should prepare by reflecting on and assessing their own performance. Additionally, by placing team emphases on the preparation questions small groups could prepare to give very specific feedback at the event.

The event should include activities that:

- look at the team's successes and challenges
- evaluate last year's objectives
- look at what individual team members contribute towards the team
- set team objectives for the forthcoming year and agree what part individuals will play in meeting those objectives.

The team event also provides the opportunity for sub-groups within the team to work together on all or part of the team's objectives.

Team appraisal can be very challenging and the team needs to guard against trying to undertake team-building activities or simply trying to resolve personal differences between team members. To be effective the event needs to be disciplined and keep focused on appraisal outcomes.

Following the event and agreeing team objectives, individual team members need to consider their development needs in relation to the objectives, their present work and aspirations. Some of this may be possible within the event but all team members must have the opportunity for a confidential discussion with the team leader.

In addition, the benefits of team appraisal are seen as:

- clarifying through agreed and shared objectives a process for achieving the desired vision
- increased participation of all team members in the work and priorities of the team
- improved interpersonal relationships.

Team appraisal in practice: a case study

Following the introduction of a trust-wide appraisal process the Head of Therapy Services at East Sussex NHS Trust approached the Learning & Development Department (authors of a revised appraisal policy advocating a flexible approach to implementing appraisal – see key scheme content outcomes in Box 7.5) for help to enhance an appraisal process already embedded into the department's culture over a 15-year period. Team appraisal was introduced into the Therapy Services Directorate and is still in place now.

This section identifies the process and key practical steps taken in introducing team appraisal to a group of senior physiotherapists.

Box 7.5 Scheme features

Extract from the appraisal policy

The recommended trust-wide appraisal system is underpinned by the following principles. It:

- allows departments to retain the positive parts of existing schemes
- allows departments to use approaches promoted by their individual professional bodies
- is an open, honest mutual communication exchange
- takes in all staff including medical
- clearly locates responsibility for appraisal with line managers
- is not a substitute for day-to-day management of performance
- is aligned to the business planning process of the trust
- provides a flexible framework for the appraisal process, not a rigid structure
- allows freedom of choice over the use of the supporting paperwork
- may use different approaches to appraisal including one-to-one, team and 360° (*see* Chapter 8)
- focuses upon measurable outcomes that are actively implemented and monitored.

There are four outcomes of the appraisal and development review process.

1 The line manager is required to retain a formal record of the appraisal process that will be kept on the confidential departmental personal file. The individual(s) being appraised must agree the record and keep a copy.
2 A personal development plan that identifies the learning needs of the staff being appraised will be sent to the HR Department to inform future education, training and development provision.
3 Details of the agreed objectives for the forthcoming year will be sent to the manager's manager to review that those objectives are in line with the overall objectives of the trust.
4 Appraisal review dates will be agreed.

To maximise flexibility no specific format for paperwork is mandatory. The objectives and personal development plan can be forwarded in writing, or by email.

Review with a more senior member of staff will be put in place to enable anyone to raise concerns about how the appraisal process has been conducted. The review will aim to resolve issues without recourse to the trust's grievance procedure.

The implementation process

An introductory event was attended by 80% of the senior physiotherapists, two senior line managers and the Head of Therapy Services supported by a facilitator. The purpose for introducing team appraisal was outlined, its relevance to achieving departmental goals clarified, the benefits to maintaining and developing services was reviewed as well as clarifying what individual team members could gain from taking part in the process.

The key benefits confirmed through discussion were:

- reviewing the role of line managers and span of control for undertaking regular appraisals
- minimising unnecessary repetition and saving time
- involving people in the process and encouraging ownership
- shared objectives and understanding of individual and collective contribution to their achievement
- encouraging staff to take responsibility for clinical and management activities
- stimulating interest in the process
- further develop team working
- encouraging initiatives and innovation
- assisting personal development
- gap analysis – identify where we are now in achieving departmental objectives and where we need to be
- learning from one another.

Inevitably the discussions identified gaps in:

- understanding and expectation of roles and responsibilities of all key players
- working boundaries related to grade, specialty, service, audit and standards.

For clarity, a working definition was agreed upon and key roles identified. The senior therapist was recognised as 'providing a clinical service with expertise' in four main roles.

1 Education.
2 Service development.
3 Management responsibilities.
4 Clinical case loads.

This framework was then adopted as a structure for identifying and agreeing objectives at further events.

From the first meeting key actions were agreed to support identifying team objectives before the second event.

- Seniors would clarify their roles and responsibilities from a specialty team and individual practitioner focus.
- Those staff who work as individual (on their own) practitioners were to form their own 'team' for this purpose.
- Management team (physiotherapy line managers plus Head of Therapy Services) were to review senior information to confirm clinical and management responsibilities.
- A second team event to take place.

The first event was effective in promoting interest in team appraisal and engaging people in the process.

An interim discussion by the management team and communicated to the seniors confirmed that the senior role comprised management and clinical components. It was decided that these components were intrinsically linked and it was considered risky to try and differentiate between the time spent separately in either element. For example writing care pathways was both a clinical and management activity. Therefore it was agreed that management tasks applied to all seniors.

The first follow-up event took place three months later. The explicit agenda was to review progress since the first event, set ground rules for the process, agree common objectives for the team and then agree a process for team and individual objectives to be set.

Box 7.6 Outline structure for the event

- Feedback from day one.
- Reprise benefits of appraisal.
- Clarify framework for the morning's work.
- Develop relationship between agreed objectives, clinical role and patient care.
- Develop common team objectives.
- Identify which team objectives groups can sign up to.
- Final discussion: what structure and support need to be in place to enable the objectives to be achieved.
- Link to appraisal process established.

Working in a cabaret-style environment, participants chose to work on clarifying specific objective areas and were then asked to validate their colleagues' work by adding to the four objective themes which metamorphosed into ten action areas.

Immediate further work was planned to clarify objectives further and select objectives for individuals/sub-teams to work on.

A key outcome was the decision that appraisal would be the framework to link clinical expertise, clinical practice, CPD and the achievement of service objectives. The appraisal process was identified as a process to help the team to review and plan.

A second follow-up event took place within four weeks at the request of the seniors. The primary agenda was to agree 'who' was going to be doing 'what', 'how' and 'when'.

Key process issues were also reviewed.

- How would objective areas be validated?
- What related activities would be required to support objective achievement?
- What process would need to be adopted to ensure objectives were progressed?
- How would the objective setting process relate to personal development planning?
- How would all team members be kept informed/involved in sub-team activities?

- What ongoing review process needed to be established to support continuous improvement in the team?

The key factors influencing the successful implementation of the process were agreed as:

- time
- sustaining patient care
- availability
- commitment
- competence
- money
- continuous improvement
- service perspective
  - inpatient
  - outpatient.

Significantly the key team objective themes were identified (Box 7.7).

Box 7.7 Significant team objective themes

Objectives outline for Senior Therapists: first draft
Overall focus: to improve patient care.

Area A: Education
To facilitate effective in-service training.

Who:

By when:

1 provide time and appropriate learning environment
2 identify staff learning needs for all grades
3 ensure equality of access to learning opportunities in terms of regularity, access and consistency
4 encourage opportunities for multi-professional learning
5 identify resources to learn: time, money, etc., and learning resources: technology, shadowing, etc.
6 develop a learning programme for the department
7 identify skills within the department team
8 set up, maintain and review recording and monitoring system of what takes place and what doesn't

To further develop external learning activities:

1 involve GPs and consultants in learning events
2 educate GPs on appropriate referral criteria.

See link with joint working below.

Area B: Service development

To take a systematic approach to planning clinical audit across the department.

Who:

By when:

1 to audit inpatient notes
2 to audit patient handouts
3 to agree a programme of specialty audits: medicine referral criteria, weekend orthopaedics service, evidence-based practice
4 to agree protocols for audits in the future

To base the working framework on agreed guidelines:

1 to identify ways to change practice using research, guidelines, frameworks, etc. (could be department-wide or specialty-specific)
2 to identify ways in which research is being used in everyday practice
3 to identify CPD requirements from improved alignment with guidelines, protocols, frameworks, etc.

To work in partnership with colleagues across the local health economy:

1 identify joint working opportunities
2 identify joint working practices
3 identify opportunities for shared learning activities.

Area C: Management

To manage the junior staff.

Who:

By when:

1 plan and organise the work
2 agree regular meetings
3 lead by example
4 provide opportunities for juniors to gain experience to supplement their knowledge base
5 review performance

To improve ways and opportunities to communicate across the whole team:

1 identify current methods of communication: what works and what doesn't
2 implement a revised structured process of communication for the team
3 identify a systematic feedback system to encourage two-way communication across the department.

To assist line managers:

1 clarify specific and joint responsibilities for managing:
   - risk management
   - health and safety
   - communication
   - payroll
   - attendance management

- IPR
- feedback

2 to effectively work together as a team
3 identify administrative requirements.

Area D: Clinical caseload

To manage the clinical caseload.

Who:

By when:

1 agree workload volumes, complexity of cases and variances
2 to manage the resource effectively to meet targets
3 to work within agreed guidelines for professional practice
4 to identify and access support mechanisms where necessary

To contribute to multidisciplinary working:

1 be proactive and raise the profile of physiotherapy in the MDT
2 to encourage opportunities for networking
3 to get 'back to the floor'
4 to agree patient outcomes and goals which are validated and part of an agreed (universal) system.

Team objectives summary plan

Area

Specific activities required

Team/Specialty/Individual

Area A
Area B
Area C
Area D
Other

Personal development plan

Personal and professional objectives

Objectives related to achieving the team objectives

Objectives for personal/professional development

Target date

The personal development plan should be sent to the Learning and Development Team to inform future education, training and development provision.

Mid-term barriers

At this point a number of barriers were identified to the smooth integration of team appraisal into the management process. These continued to be a feature until the team appraisal process became mainstreamed into the culture of the team 18 months down the line.

The general objectives of getting team objectives on team meeting agendas and general communication were found to be a challenge – explicit links between new processes and old working habits needed to be challenged.

Meeting with the senior line managers became disjointed. There was a lack of integration of the team appraisal process into the normal management processes of the department; the result was duplication of activity and in some instances potential for conflict. The challenge of changing boundaries and delegating responsibilities and yet maintaining that delicate balance of freedom and control became quite blurred.

Meetings of the sub-teams generated a lot of 'behind the scenes' activity. However, there were missed opportunities for joined-up thinking across the themes and for wider communication across the physiotherapy team.

A final whole team review workshop was held six months later. (This was undoubtedly the most exciting workshop of the process.) The four sub-teams came prepared to present on progress to date, the steps they took, identifying what had worked and what had not, what the planned next steps were and what further help, if any, was required.

The room was alive as individual, sub-team and whole team discussions took place about changes, services, standards, improvements, etc.

As a result of this event further actions were agreed.

- Structured communication processes put in place – regular meetings, revised meeting format, style, involvement and output. Team objectives to be a standing item on meeting agendas.
- A summary of progress to be produced and experiences shared (which has informed this case study).
- Monthly meetings to be established to align the team appraisal process with the management process.

The way ahead for the team included an ongoing team-wide review process and a clear short-term agenda to improve:

- communication
- integration
- personal development
- decision-making processes
- explicit levels of authority
- management responsibilities vs being a manager
- management and leadership skills development.

The final link: personal development planning

Once the team service objectives were identified, the line managers supplemented the objective setting process with individual (30 minute) discussions which related personal development needs to current, expected and developmental performance. Further clarification was required where some service objectives needed to be shared by all seniors and this was confirmed through the one-to-one sessions. Ensuring everyone remained engaged in the team achievement of objectives became a monitoring role for the line managers.

Conclusion

A significant investment was made in time to engage and commit the team to the revised process. Much valuable organisational learning took place as the process evolved. Meaningful objectives and priorities were achieved in a co-operative and partnership way. The senior roles have been enhanced and their management responsibilities fulfilled. Our new challenge is establishing what impact the *Agenda for Change* process will have on this approach.

Measuring the impact

The review process instigated to review the effectiveness of the team appraisal process is a useful approach to apply to any locally implemented scheme. As identified earlier, the National Staff Attitude survey now collects quantitative and qualitative data on appraisal. To assess locally how effective the implementation of an appraisal scheme is, the following measures could be put in place.

Short-term measures could include:

- completion rate of forms
- deployment could be benchmarked against the initial analysis from this review process
- actions generated from the appraisal process itself
- success in achieving short-term goals
- the general attitude and value of the appraisal approach through random or systematic evaluation
- impact on staff attitude surveys.

Long-term measures could include:

- effective use of development resources
- reviewing organisational performance
- staff retention rates
- staff turnover rates
- sickness and absence rates
- delivery against long-term development targets.

The editors wish to acknowledge with thanks the work of the Eastbourne physiotherapy team for the case study outlined in this chapter.

References

1   Department of Health. *A First Class Service: quality in the new NHS*. London: Department of Health; 1998.
2   NHS Executive. *Working Together: securing a quality workforce for the NHS*. London: NHS Executive; 1998.

3 Borril C, West M. In: *Effective Human Resource Management and Patient Mortality*. Birmingham: Aston University; 2002.
4 NHSME. *IPR Training Knowledge Book*. London: NHSME; 1986.
5 Long P. *Performance Appraisal Revisited*. London: IPM; 1986.
6 Department of Health. *Agenda for Change*. London: Stationery Office; 2004.
7 Department of Health. *The NHS Knowledge and Skills Framework and the Development Review Process*. London: Stationery Office; 2004.

Bibliography

Abbot V, Powell D. *Competency Based Appraisal Systems: a survey report*; 1997.

Appraisal Information for East Sussex Hospitals NHS Trust (2003–2005) – with a debt of gratitude to Bob Dibley, Learning and Development Manager.

Audit Commission. *The Doctor's Tale Continued*. London: HMSO; 1996.

BAMM. *Appraisal In Action*. London: BAMM; 1999.

BMA. *Appraisal for Senior Hospital Doctors*. London: BMA; 1998.

Brotherton P. Candid feedback spurs changes in culture. *HRM Magazine*. 1996; **May**.

Eastbourne Hospitals Trust. *Openness, Involvement and Partnership – an action plan*. Eastbourne: Eastbourne Hospitals Trust; 2000.

Fletcher C. *Appraisal: routes to improved performance*. 2nd edn. London: IPD; 1997.

Harrington HJ. Performance improvement: was W Edwards Deming wrong? *TQM Magazine*. 1999; **10**(4): 230–37.

NHS Executive. *The Vital Connection: an equalities framework for the NHS*. London: NHS Executives 2000.

NHS Executive. *Working Together: securing a quality workforce for the NHS*. London: NHS Executive; 1998.

Raven J. Professional appraisal in nurse education: findings of a pilot study. *CPD Magazine*. 1999; **2**.

Weightman J. *Managing People in the Health Service*. London: IPD; 1996.

Chapter 8

Appraisal: 360° feedback

Simon and Sheena Loveday

When we were asked to write this chapter, our first reaction was, 'why us?'. The reason was a session one of us had given on this topic at an NHS leadership training event. The person who put us forward for this chapter had been a participant on the programme. She had come into the session feeling, 'I couldn't possibly do this – much too scary'. She left feeling, 'This feels well worth while – and I think I could do it'. If readers of this chapter leave with the same feeling, then our time in writing it will have been well spent.

Introduction: what is 360° feedback? And what is the point of gathering it?

360° feedback is simply a method for gathering information from those around you, about the effectiveness of your behaviour. 'Feedback' refers to a response or reaction; '360°' indicates that it goes right round the compass to cover all angles on you and what you do, from your boss above you, through your peers beside you, to your reports below you in the organisational tree. When you set out to gather 360° feedback, you are simply asking those most affected by your behaviour to tell you how your behaviour impacts upon them, what messages (intentional or unintentional) you are sending, what works well – and what needs improving.

Put as simply as that, it is perhaps strange that we don't use the technique more often. After all, we interact with others every day, and our behaviour affects them constantly. The same is true in reverse: others' behaviour affects us all the time, and sometimes we long for the opportunity to encourage them to do more of what works – or to find ways to stop them doing what doesn't work. Organisations use it a lot in the form of questionnaires and satisfaction surveys; car manufacturers, garages, supermarkets, hotels, local councils, even training providers, are constantly asking us whether we are happy with what they do. Feedback (in the sense we are using here) is now a fact of life. And given that our behaviour is the only tool we have for influencing others, it would be strange if we didn't invest some serious time in finding out whether the tool is working properly.

However, most of us also have a degree of apprehension in asking others for feedback – particularly such 'significant others' as boss, peers, reports, and customers (or patients). One apprehension is about the possibility of 'bad news' – what if they don't like the way we behave towards them? Worse, what if they don't like who we are? How will we face them at work when we know that?

Curiously, however, another apprehension is about good news. The English reluctance to confront feelings directly means that direct praise can be as embarrassing as direct criticism. So even getting good feedback and enthusiastic affirmation of what we do can still be uncomfortable!

How might we overcome this reluctance?

A good way, we would suggest, is to reframe the whole concept of 360° feedback. Its parenthood is stern. Its father is appraisal – a manager assessing and judging the effectiveness of the work of a member of their staff. Its mother, born perhaps 30 years ago, is upward appraisal – direct reports assessing and judging the effectiveness of the person who manages them. But 360° feedback at its best is different from both its parents. This difference is best thought of in three ways.

1   As a process, not the one-off annual event of appraisal.
2   To remember that it is about development, not about assessment. Apart from your boss, those whom you ask for feedback won't have power over you or over your salary.
3   This one grows from the first two – not as a method of judging your effectiveness, but rather as a way of involving others in your development. Used correctly, 360° feedback gives others the chance to help you be more effective, to grow, and to develop. And most of your respondents will be pleased to be asked – and appreciative of the chance to be involved in this process.

So why use this process?

The most important question is the initial one: Why do you want feedback? What do you want feedback about?

There can be a variety of reasons. Perhaps you are going for a promotion, or for a development opportunity such as a leadership workshop, and want to check out your performance in your current role. Perhaps you lead a team and want to hear both from them and from your boss what you do that works, and what you could do better. Perhaps you want to involve customers, peers, service users, or patients in the process. Perhaps you are unsure of what your strengths are. Perhaps you are very well aware of some aspects of your behaviour that get in the way – but you are working on them, and want to know if those aspects are still a problem. Perhaps you have never 'looked in the mirror' in this way before, and feel that it is time you did a reality check. And perhaps you feel that it is important to consult others because they are on the receiving end of what you do, and you want to show them that you take their views seriously.

The great benefit of the 360° process is the reality check – the ability to 'see ourselves as others see us'. But it is not without its risks. One risk is outside you – that some of the recipients might use it as an opportunity to offload on you grudges and grievances that are not really yours at all, but belong to the organisation. Another 'outside' risk is that people will tell you what they think you want to hear. But the principal risk is inside you – that you will hear something that you are unable or unwilling to receive. If you don't want, or don't feel strong enough, or don't feel ready, to hear others' views, the answer is simple: don't ask. Don't embark on the process until you feel ready to take it on.

So, as in most things, there can be 'enemies without' and 'enemies within'. How can we tackle these?

First, it is helpful to ask yourself, 'is there anything about me, or the way I receive comments, that could make people reluctant to be honest with me? Am I very sensitive to criticism? How ready will others be to speak their minds?'. Second, it is well to ask yourself how your manager will respond: will their comments be constructive, or will they just take it as an opportunity to dwell on any weaknesses they see? And thirdly, think about the context around you. Is now the right moment for the exercise? Will your respondents give it their full attention? Will they see it for what it is, or will they find some sinister ulterior motive in it? Is the organisation one in which it is possible for staff and colleagues to speak honestly and directly? Again, if you're not sure of the answers to these questions, you need to explore further before you launch in.

Putting it into practice: choosing the right method

The first question is always, 'what sort of data do you want?'. That will always determine the kind of questions you ask. You might want to know how you perform against a set of competencies (e.g. the Leadership Qualities Framework, or a more general leadership or managerial competency framework). You might want to know what you need to do in order to maximise your chances of promotion. You might want to know how you're doing as a team leader – as a team member – as a colleague – as an AHP practitioner – as a GP. You might simply be interested in your own development for its own sake.

When you start to look at the range of 360° tools and instruments on the market you will be amazed. (A recent search on Google threw up 34 900 results.) There are huge numbers, and great complexity. A good selection principle is to remember when you filled in a feedback form for someone else. How easy was it? How quick? How satisfying? At the end, did you feel you had said what you wanted to say, or were your answers cramped and constrained by the format of the questions? There are a number of questionnaires which look impressive in their range and numerical thoroughness, but which suffer from two problems. The first is 'respondent fatigue' – which sets in relatively quickly! And the second is spurious precision. A lot of questionnaires ask for number scores and will add, average, and differentiate them in clever ways but it is difficult to know what weight to put on the original scores. If you ask to be rated on a 1–5 scale, someone with low expectations may rate you at 5 because you are better than they expected. Someone else may rate you at only 4 because they never give 5s. And a third respondent may rate you at only 2 because they are fed up with managers (or GPs, or consultants, or whatever category you fall into) and all they want is an excuse to work off their frustration. How do you add up these incompatible ratings and get a meaningful average? So, be wary of complexity for its own sake.

A good rule of thumb is:

- ask only the questions that matter to you in your current situation
- ask both for numbers and for comments (quantitative and qualitative data)
- stick to words that will have meaning for your respondents
- end with an open-ended question

and above all:

- keep it short!

How to gather the feedback

You have a number of choices. Do you want the comments to be made in writing, or given to you face to face? (A good combination is to use both: ask people to complete a questionnaire, then to talk it through with you. For more on this, see 'Receiving the feedback' below.)

If in writing, do you want hard copy, or email? Email is quick and easy and people like it; the response rate is usually better. But some of your respondents may not have access to it, and there may be security or confidentiality issues.

If entirely face to face without anything in writing, you must take notes and, very importantly, you must check them back with the respondent at the end of the session to ensure that what you heard is really what they said.

You may feel that the people – or the culture – aren't ready for the openness of direct feedback, and that you will get a better and more honest response if you ask for anonymous comments, so that respondents feel more free to speak their minds – and so that you feel more confidence in positive comments. And since it will be difficult for respondents to maintain that anonymity if comments come direct to you (you'll often recognise handwriting, and it's hard to send an anonymous email!), then you can ask a third party to collect and collate comments for you. This of course is where external providers come in. If you go to an external provider, make sure that you look at a sample profile to see how they treat the data. Two questions worth asking are, do they include all the raw data? (They should. It's the most powerful part.) And do they summarise the salient points for you – and if so, how? (Be sceptical of so-called 'intelligent systems' that produce text reports. Systems they may be, but they aren't always very intelligent.)

Don't just ask others for their scores and comments – enter yours on the questionnaire as well. (If nothing else, it will tell you whether the questionnaire is easy and practical to complete, or the reverse.) Self-assessment is interesting for its own sake, but its primary value is to give you a reference point when you're reading respondents' scores and comments. If you think you're weak in a certain area and they do too, then at least your reality matches theirs. If your views and theirs don't match, you've learned something worth knowing – and better still, something worth investigating.

Further points to look out for in questionnaire design? On the numerical side, our experience is that a scale of 1–5 is best; ensure that people know whether 1 is low or high (mark it on every page). Give respondents the option of leaving a blank or ticking a 'Don't know' box if they want to – otherwise you will not be able to tell whether a 3 is a genuine middle score, or a way of saying that there is not enough evidence either way.

What questions to ask

As usual, it depends on what answers you want! We can split this into four possibilities. The first is to use a standard 360° questionnaire, either one current in your organisation, or a commercially available one. This has the advantage of saving you a lot of work; it will probably be quite thorough and wide-ranging; and it may give you some useful comparative data against a benchmark of other organisations. On the downside, it may not ask quite the questions you want answered, it won't use precisely the language of your organisation – and you may have to pay for it.

A second option, if your organisation has a list of competencies that are applicable to your role, is to simply send round that list and ask people to rate you against each competency on a 1–5 scale. That is again quite labour-saving (for you), it is specific to your organisation, and it is respectful of the fact that the organisation has put time and money into developing the competencies. The biggest disadvantages are, first, that there are sometimes quite a lot of competencies – and second, that many competencies appear only distantly related to the real world of work, with the result that respondents don't find it very easy to write genuine answers that express what they want to say. Of how many of your colleagues could you say that they;

> Accurately interpret the underlying causes of others' behaviour, recognising their needs, concerns, and feelings whether expressed or implicit?

Would you want to rate a colleague for:

> Understands and conveys the mission and vision of the organisation with passion and conviction?

(Indeed, would you want to work with anyone like that?) The Leadership Qualities Framework is not always beyond reproach here.

If it is your leadership qualities and potential that you want to explore, you might try the approach suggested by Pedler and Burgoyne in their *Manager's Guide to Self-Development*. They put forward seven criteria for effective leadership – and offer a simple questionnaire which asks respondents not only to rate you, but to rate the importance of each quality. You may not find the seven criteria completely convincing but what the method does provide is a simple grid which enables you to identify at a glance the areas where your respondents feel you need to focus.

A third option, as we have seen, is to design your own questionnaire focusing on what you want to find out. An elegant preliminary to this is to ask your respondents – your patients, for example, or the members of your team – what qualities are important to them, what they are looking for from you, and then to use these questions, so that they have in effect designed the questionnaire that they will then be asked to respond to. This method has a lot to recommend it!

With all three methods, it depends on how much information you want. (That's one reason why it's a good idea to fill out the questionnaire yourself before you give it to others.) If you want a lot of information, encourage your respondents to provide examples by every question. But whatever method you use, it's always a good idea to provide an opportunity for participants to write what they want to say – rather than what you want to ask. A simple and well-proven way to do this is to use the A4 page suggested below (*see* Box 8.1): the page can go either at the start or the finish of the questionnaire.

> **Box 8.1 Preliminary questionnaire**
>
> Pen Picture: what words or phrases would you use to describe this person?
>   What do you see as their special strengths? What qualities do they bring to their job?
>   [Optional, if you are exploring your further career development] How do you see their future in your organisation?
>   In order to be at their most effective, is there anything they should do differently?

We suggested that there were four options. The fourth option is simply to use the page above on its own. It is quick and easy for respondents to complete, and for you or your data-collector to process; and its simplicity not only increases the likelihood of a response, but also ensures that the big issues will leap off the page. Moreover they will be phrased in the respondents' own words. Those are not inconsiderable advantages!

Who (and how many) to ask

The first and best rule is, 'ask people whose opinions you respect'. If you aren't going to listen to the answer, don't bother to ask the question. By definition, 360° feedback has some givens in it: upwards, sideways, downwards. But there is often some choice in that. If you do have a choice, don't feel that you have to 'seek balance' by going out of your way to include someone who you know dislikes you or has a low opinion of you. That isn't balance. That's tokenism, and it allows you to say, 'I know where that comment comes from – and I don't have to pay attention to it because they always say that about me'. Go for people you can learn from: people you respect, and who know you well enough for their opinions and judgements to matter to you. They may or may not dislike you or be in conflict with you; what matters is that you value what they say. And it doesn't have to be people who have known you a long time. It can equally be people who haven't been in your team or your work environment for long, so that what you are learning is how you come across at first impression.

A good second rule is to look at your important relationships – the ones that repay an investment of time and energy. That may include clients or key internal customers; it may also include your secretary or PA.

Don't be put off by closeness. By all means ask work colleagues who are also friends (as long as you know that friendship won't get in the way of honesty). If it's a personal topic you're interested in, feel free to ask friends outside work, and even partners or close family. But don't only ask the people you get on with. Be prepared to ask those you don't get on with too. Just stick to the two basic rules above: important relationships, and opinions you will respect.

A final point about numbers. A lot of the commercial questionnaires advise you to ask widely – up to 12 or 14 people. Part of the reason is because they assume there will be a wide drop-out rate, but there is also an assumption that more data mean a better result. We would challenge that assumption. In our view, this exercise is about finding the key points that you need to work on in order to be more effective – and more information is as likely to confuse the issue as it is to clarify it. We would suggest six to eight is an ideal number – and aim for at least an 80% return rate. Which brings us on to briefing.

Briefing your respondents

A good starting point, once again, is to think of yourself as a respondent. Which will motivate you more, make you feel more important and valued – and increase the likelihood of your giving quality feedback: a visit from a colleague to ask for your help and explain the reasons or an email with an attachment? Most people respond better to the first, and that is the method we will advocate here. If you are going to brief your respondents, it's probably worth booking a few minutes with them – the middle of a busy office is not a good place – and ensuring that you can find a place where you can both talk freely and without disturbance. The process need not take long, but will probably need to cover:

- explaining why you are seeking feedback at all
- explaining why you have chosen that particular person
- giving them permission to speak freely (asking for some balance between support and challenge is a good way to do this)
- explaining the sequence of events and what is expected of them (is it anonymous? who do they return the form to? how will it be processed? and so on)
- clarifying the timescale
- asking for any questions or uncertainties on their part.

Finally, and most importantly:

- thanking them in advance for their help.

It is perfectly possible to put all this in a letter, email, or phone call but face to face works best and sends out the message that you value the person and have chosen them personally.

Using other instruments

One of the ways you can help respondents to give you good feedback is to identify the points that give you concern. Are you worried that you might be a bit too pushy? Not pushy enough? Over-concerned with detail? Not sufficiently concerned with detail? The answer is simply to ask: 'I'd particularly like feedback on whether I've got the right balance with detail/firmness/pace' – or whatever your concern is.

This process can be sharpened and focused by the use of personality questionnaires. Most questionnaires give you a view of what you are like at your best – and what you are like at your worst! The one we will touch on here is the Belbin Team Role questionnaire, which is available on the web at www.belbin.com for a modest fee. R Meredith Belbin, an occupational psychologist, designed this questionnaire in the 1980s as result of research carried out at Henley Management College. He and his research colleagues identified eight team roles (since expanded to nine) which are essential if a team is to function properly. All of us will have a preference for a particular team role. Belbin's descriptions identify for

Table 8.1 Belbin Shaper role

Strength (key quality they bring to the team)	Allowable weakness (how they may irritate other team members)
Shaper Dynamic, outgoing, competitive. Challenges, pressurises, finds ways round obstacles. Drives team to finish first.	Prone to impatience (which may or may not be successfully contained!).

each team role a key contribution which people with that preference bring to the team – but also what he delightfully calls an 'allowable weakness', which is of course the same strength, but overdone. A good example is what he calls the Shaper role – the tough, driving leader who helps the team to strive for excellence, and without whom the team too easily settles for second best. Table 8.1 shows what Belbin says about the Shaper role.

If you take the questionnaire and find out that your preferred role is indeed Shaper, then you can easily add that description to your briefing, asking whether your respondents see either positive or negative signs of that characteristic in you – and whether the negative side is a concern to them. (Remember that they may well see the weakness, but be prepared to put up with it on the grounds that the benefits outweigh the costs. It is, after all, in Belbin's term, 'allowable'!)

A general principle of any exercise of this kind is that when personality characteristics are openly acknowledged, they are much easier to deal with. Perfection isn't given to many human beings: honesty is.

Receiving the feedback

So you have decided an area to explore, selected a method, and chosen and briefed your respondents. How will you go about receiving the feedback?

Receiving written feedback

Most feedback is received in writing – either 'raw', or summarised into a report. The first thing to say is that feedback about ourselves is amazingly difficult to hear and take in clearly. It is sometimes said that feedback is like a torch: when we point it at others we see them more clearly, but when it is pointed at us, it blinds us and prevents us from seeing anything at all. So don't expect to absorb it all at once: sleep on it first.

A good way to come back to it and process it is to write a little grid that looks like Figure 8.1, using two axes: expected/unexpected, and positive/negative (or corrective). (There are other ways to do this but this will do for now.)

These four boxes can tell you a great deal. Is there nothing much in any of the boxes? Perhaps your respondents don't feel confident (or involved) enough to give you much feedback. Is there a lot in the top two boxes? (Remember to have a look at your self-assessments to see what you wrote about yourself before you heard others' views.) If there is, then your self-image doesn't entirely match reality. Is there a lot in Box 4? Then you have had some useful confirmation that

1 Unexpected corrective feedback	2 Unexpected positive feedback
3 Expected corrective feedback	4 Expected positive feedback

Figure 8.1 Feedback grid

you are on the right track. Or is there a lot in Box 1? Then you really do have some work to do – and some conversations to have.

The final part of this written 'dialogue with yourself' is to complete a final box (*see* Box 8.2).

Box 8.2 Self-dialogue

Areas I need to develop

Actions I need to take

People I need to talk to

Receiving feedback – or checking it out – face to face

It may be that you have the opportunity to talk through some of your feedback face to face. We started this chapter by suggesting that:

> 360° feedback is simply a method for gathering information from those around you, about the effectiveness of your behaviour.

That is a good frame of mind in which to approach a face-to-face session, whether it is new information, or checking out what you have already heard: an attitude of detached curiosity, in which both giver and receiver are engaged in a joint project.

Some points here are obvious: set aside enough time – up to an hour if possible; find a quiet place; keep an open mind; take notes. Some are less obvious. One is, always ask for evidence:

> You say I'm very effective as a leader. What is it that I do that makes you say that? Where have you seen me be effective?

> You say that I'm not always sensitive to others' needs and feelings. What is it that I do that makes you say that? Where have you seen this happen?

A second way of drawing out information is to use the formula, 'and is there anything else?'.

Third, give permission to your respondent to speak openly – not just by explicitly inviting open feedback, but also by offering specific ways into that feedback:

> I've had comments that I can be a bit short-tempered and that's something I'd particularly like to check out.

> I am working on being simpler and clearer and I'd like your views on whether that's succeeding.

People with my Myers Briggs Type Indicator (MBTI) can find it a bit difficult to share their thinking with others, and I'd like to find out whether that's causing a problem. (MBTI, *see* Chapter 9)

Fourth, remember that you're on the same side as your respondent: what they're giving you is what you've asked for, so don't interrupt, contradict or try to justify yourself or your behaviour. (We defined feedback earlier as 'a way of involving others in your development'.) You don't have to act on what they say – but the least you can do is to hear it, explore it, and take note of it. How you receive feedback will determine whether you go on getting it!

So, end by thanking them – and by asking them if you can come back to them with any questions later. Very few people will say no.

So what next – how do you follow up?

We suggested in a previous section that you would do well to list the areas you need to develop; the actions you need to take; and – crucially – the people you need to talk to. If the exercise has been worth undertaking, it is surely worth sharing the results with your manager (given that they were involved anyway). One action you will certainly want to carry out is to thank those who responded to your request; one action you might want to take is to share with them the key points from your feedback, and the actions you are taking as a result. You might ask respondents if they are willing to give you continuing help with your development points:

I'm working on this area and would like to know how I'm doing . . . if you see me do this please tell me.

And this shouldn't be a one-off; a note in your diary to check things three months, or even a year, later will pay dividends ('a way of involving others in your development . . .').

Should you run the questionnaire again? It might seem a good idea, but we would advise caution here. Questionnaires are subjective and interactive. In practice this means that respondents compare you with their expectations of you. The first time round, this is new data. But a re-run of a questionnaire means that their expectations will have changed. It is not unusual for second-time-round scores to be *lower* rather than higher – not because the questioner is less effective, but because participants are sensitised, and conditioned to expect more. So by all means go round and ask but be wary about a simple re-run.

Finally, a familiar pattern in human nature, at least in British nature, is to focus on what we do badly and need to do less of. But another way of looking at feedback is to focus on what we do well and need to do more of. It may be that the feedback has highlighted certain strengths and a need to do them more. We should not forget the message implicit in the Belbin questionnaire, that each team role has strengths and weaknesses, but that the strengths and the weaknesses are closely bound up, and that the weaknesses are 'allowable'. So if you have had some positive feedback – particularly if it was unexpectedly positive – you might give yourself a moment of praise!

References

1   Pedler J, Burgoyne M. *Manager's Guide to Self-Development*. London: McGraw Hill; 1998/2001.
2   The Belbin questionnaire is available online at www.belbin.com.
3   Belbin RM. *Management Teams: why they succeed or fail*. Oxford: Heinemann; 1981.

Chapter 9

Using the Myers Briggs Type Indicator within the Allied Health Professions

Simon and Sheena Loveday

Introduction

This chapter is about the Myers Briggs Type Indicator (MBTI),[1] a personality or 'psychometric' questionnaire widely used in business, in healthcare, and in personal development. The chapter sets out to explain what the MBTI is, how it can be useful to you, and how to learn more about it.

The authors of this chapter are MBTI enthusiasts and use it both inside and outside work. However, we are not setting out to seek converts. Our hope is that you will read this chapter with an open mind, but not so open that your brain falls out! By all means be sceptical: you need to find out whether this is a method and an approach that will work for you and we welcome a readiness to challenge and question. But please, if your mind is closed already, read no further. We don't expect to convince you on the basis of one article!

The purpose of this chapter is to introduce the MBTI to AHPs and to give them an idea of how it can help them:

- to understand themselves better
- to value themselves and others more
- to get the best from themselves and others
- to become more effective in their working relationships.

Five scenarios

How might you know you're achieving these objectives? If the MBTI is the answer, what is the question? Here are five scenarios. If any of them fit – read on.

1   You have reached a decision point in your career. You have to choose between continuing in a specialist role, or becoming a generalist. The financial and promotion aspects point clearly in one direction – but your instincts are set in the other. How could you get a better understanding of your reservations in this matter?

2   You work closely with a colleague. At first you really liked their quiet, thoughtful, undemonstrative style. But now it is beginning to drive you mad. The more you push for responses from them, the less you get. What can you do?

3   You are a GP. One of your recent consultations involved a very rare complaint – you have never seen one outside a textbook. You successfully identified the

problem and were successful in insisting that the patient take appropriate action. Now, to your dismay, you hear that the patient has lodged a complaint against you! What has gone wrong?

4   You work as part of a practice team. The team has agreed its targets and objectives at the start of the year and set them out clearly in a schedule – but you seem to be the only one of your colleagues who is attending to them. In previous years your colleagues have 'got there' fine in the end, but the uncertainty, and their lack of concern, are driving you crazy. How can you and they come to some kind of agreed style?

5   Mostly you handle work pressures pretty well – but sometimes you find yourself responding in a way that seems completely out of character. How can you prevent this happening again? And is there a way you and your colleagues can see it coming next time, and either guard against it, or minimise its impact?

Background to the indicator

The MBTI is a personality test. Its underlying principles derive from the work of Carl Jung (1875–1961),[2,3] the brilliant Swiss psychologist and philosopher who coined, among other things, the terms 'extravert' and 'introvert'. Jung was for a number of years a close associate of Sigmund Freud, but Freud's insistence on the need for a close adherence to his beliefs and assumptions led to a breakdown of the relationship in 1911–12. This was a great shock to Jung and he spent much of the war years – Switzerland of course being neutral – in trying to work out how two people could differ fundamentally, and yet still 'both be right'. The result of that was *Psychological Types*. Three of the four dimensions of the Indicator were set out in that book. It was translated into English in 1923 and read by an American woman with a strong interest in character and personality – Katharine Briggs – and her daughter Isabel Myers. When America entered the Second World War in 1942, Isabel and Katharine turned to Jung's work for two reasons: first, to find an instrument that would help people find their niche in the turmoil of conscription and war work; and secondly, from a more idealistic drive closely related to Jung's, to find a way to understand and respect others, or in a phrase that became a beacon for Isabel, to 'value difference'.

The resulting questionnaire (of which more below) went through 30 years of research before becoming available to the general public in 1975. The research base is huge and growing and its validity has been tested and established worldwide. Over three million people take it in English each year and it is now available in 15 languages.

Before explaining what it *is*, we should explain clearly what it *isn't*. It doesn't measure ability; it doesn't measure sanity (or insanity); and it shouldn't be used (on its own at least) for selection. So what does it do?

Type and preference

The basic theories of the Indicator are built round the concepts of *type* and *preference*. The simplest way to illustrate this is to invite you to write your name – but with your wrong hand. When people describe what this is like, they tend to come up with words like 'awkward . . . difficult . . . takes concentration . . . slow . . .

shaky'. Sometimes it makes them cross – 'why am I doing this when I can do it perfectly well with the other hand?' – or insecure and anxious. Sometimes, on the other hand, they find it an enjoyable challenge, even fun.

And the result? A frequent comment is that it looks 'like a child's writing'. Often people notice too that they have written very big, which in turn makes it almost exaggeratedly clear.

Doing this exercise illustrates a key way in which MBTI theory is different from most psychological theories. Most personality tests are based on a central core of normal behaviour – confidence, sociability, openness, optimism, and so on. These characteristics of personality, known as traits, are distributed along a normal distribution curve: put differently, most people are in the middle. (That's why they're normal.) People with too little or too much of the trait, those who deviate from the norm, are different – or deviant. At the extremes, you don't want to employ someone like that and that's why personality tests can be very useful in selection.

But handwriting is different. We have a left hand and a right hand – and in the UK at least, it is perfectly valid to use either to write with. But almost everyone develops a preference, very early in life, which leads them to specialise in one or the other. We may use different hands for different things but we very seldom hesitate when it comes to picking up a pen. Either/or preferences of this kind, as opposed to 'too much/too little' theories illustrated earlier, are what psychologists mean when they talk about 'type'. And this approach has four important consequences.

1 That it's OK to have clear preferences: you can't 'prefer both'.
2 That both preferences are of equal value. Despite what some countries still teach in their schools, the left hand works just as well as the right hand.
3 That, just as you have a 'right hand', so you will have a 'wrong hand' – a less preferred style of behaviour. And when you use that style – when shy people try to be more assertive, or cool and distant people try to get all warm and friendly – you will probably do it rather badly, at least to start with, and above all overdo it. That's not surprising: like your wrong-handed writing, it has been lying unused and undeveloped inside you for years, indeed since your childhood.
4 That you *can* do it. People may not *want* to write with their wrong hand but everyone can do it. With practice you would get better, to the point where perhaps others didn't know it was not your usual hand (though you, of course, would). And it might even be fun!

The four dimensions of type

Jung's theory of psychological type posits that there are a number of brain functions that are binary, like a light switch. We can do one or the other – but we can't do them at the same time. In this, they are like left- and right-handedness. And in the same way, we develop a preference for one, and leave the other undeveloped.

The first of these dimensions – the E/I dimension – is about energy. People who get their energy from the outer world of people and things, Jung called extraverts – literally, 'turned outwards'. A preference of this kind tends to lead people to have:

- a preference for action
- a tendency to breadth, to knowing a little about a lot
- a need to do their thinking outwardly, by talking things over
- an open, 'WYSIWYG' personality – what you see is what you get!

Of course, they can do the opposite but it will drain their energy, and feel like hard work.

Contrasting with them are 'introverts'. Introversion has for many years had a bad press (there is a famous if untraceable story about a comment heard in an American supermarket queue, 'My daughter used to be an introvert, but she's better now'). But the term 'introversion' merely means that your energy is turned, and tuned, to the inner world of thoughts and concepts, so that:

- you will feel most at home in your inner life
- your strengths will lie in deep reflection rather than quick action, and you will usually be more of a specialist, knowing 'a lot about a little' (or having few friends, but knowing them very well)
- you will typically keep something of yourself in reserve
- in order to give of your best, others will need to allow you time to think things over – to consult your inner sources of judgement and experience and to pay attention to what they say.

Of course, introverts can and do extravert but it drains their energy, and can leave them with nothing to spare for social interaction at the end of the day.

The second dimension, the S/N scale, is about how we take in information. When we use our Sensing function, we rely on the evidence from our senses – we take in what is there, what is available to our five senses. People with a well-developed preference for Sensing will tend to:

- see what is, accept reality as it is
- enjoy the material side of life
- be realistic, practical, comfortable with detail
- adapt existing things
- focus on the past (because it is real and has really happened) and the present (because it is really happening now)
- ask 'what' question: 'what needs to be done? what do you want me to do?'.

The contrasting way of taking in information is through possibilities, connections, meanings, relationships, patterns – in essence, not seeing how things are, but how things might be. (It is sometimes said that 'scientists see what everyone has seen, but notice what nobody has noticed', and that ability to make connections and draw conclusions is characteristic of Intuition as the term is used here.) People with a well-developed preference for Intuition (it is always shortened to N to avoid confusion with I for Introversion) are likely to:

- see what might be, question reality
- be visionary, speculative, look beyond the present and the given
- seek out 'big picture' solutions and explanations
- invent new things
- focus on the future (because it hasn't happened yet and so gives plenty of scope)
- ask 'why' questions: 'Why are we doing this? Why does it have to be like this?'.

The third dimension is the T/F scale – Thinking and Feeling. This scale examines how we make decisions. Jung argued that there are two perfectly rational, but entirely separate, ways of reaching decisions. (The terms are used here in quite a special sense: 'thinkers' don't necessarily think better, and 'feelers' don't necessarily feel more.) When you use your Thinking function to make a decision, you use logical principles, you weigh things up carefully – even to the point of counting the 'for' and 'against' arguments – and you remain impersonal. If you have feelings, you seek to discount them: 'I try not to act according to feelings unless there is a rational explanation for them' (Thinking type quoted in Bayne, 1995). Thinking seeks to fit the world, and our experiences, into a logical order. And its ultimate goal – even if there is a price to pay for it – is truth.

The Feeling function reaches decisions differently – with reference to values and beliefs. What is the most important value at stake in a decision? What is the right thing to do? Your guide is values and beliefs – sometimes accessed almost by instinct rather than by a process that you can spell out and make explicit. The Feeling function emphasises relationship and connection (rather than the detachment which is a key value for the Thinking function). Feeling seeks to fit the world, and our experiences, into a moral order. And the prime goal of feeling – even if there is a price to pay for it – is harmony.

The three dimensions that we have looked at so far are those that Jung himself identified in *Psychological Types*. But Isabel and Katharine added a fourth, based on earlier research by Katharine. This is the J/P scale – Judging and Perceiving – and it identifies how we like to live our outer lives. (This, incidentally, is the scale which often plays out most visibly in family life!) People with a Judging preference seek closure; they wish their lives were organised, planned and controlled, they like the comfort of getting things decided and settled, they enjoy having dates in the diary so that they know where they will be and what they will be doing well into the future, thus minimising uncertainty. Not surprisingly, a lot of Js are managers in organisations: after all, they like things to be . . .organised! They are usually great list-makers – not just making lists, but enjoying the sensuous pleasure of crossing things off them as they get done. If you want to keep a Judging type happy, remember their motto: No surprises!

People with a Perceiving preference look across at Judging types and think . . .how sad! Get a life! The Perceiving preference is for incoming information – for leaving things open as long as possible – for curiosity, spontaneity, variety, trying things out to see if you like them. (Tigger's exploratory approach to diet in *Winnie the Pooh* is a perfect example of Perceiving in action.) Judging types can make themselves adapt; Perceiving types naturally prefer adaptability and flexibility. The structure that gives Judging types confidence and security is experienced by Perceiving types as a constraint and a prison: Don't tie me down! And the readiness of Perceiving types to leave things to the last minute – because that's the only way it is possible to guarantee having the maximum amount of information – is seen by Judging types as disorganisation and procrastination.

The linkages with family life are most obvious here: Perceiving children leaving their homework to the last minute, to the dismay of their Judging parents; the Judging partner wanting their week – or their holiday – carefully structured with every day filled, while the Perceiving partner wants to leave things open and 'see how I feel on the day'; the Judging partner sustained by lists, the Perceiving partner watching with puzzled amusement.

How do these four preferences play out in the daily reality of work and home life? The first thing to say is that they are preferences, not rigid rules: we all use all the behavioural styles, and indeed the ability to work outside our preferred style is a mark of maturity and the fully developed personality. But to be able to use a less preferred style, is not the same as preferring that style. Our preferred style is like our home – it's where we feel safe and comfortable. We don't spend all our time there, but we need to know where it is.

The second point to make is that these preferences don't work in isolation. Like ingredients in a menu, they work together to produce a whole person. There are 16 possible combinations of the four letters. If we take four at random – Introversion, Sensing, Thinking, and Judging – we come up with the ISTJ type.

- Introversion provides reflection and depth.
- Sensing provides realism and an eye for detail.
- Thinking provides logic and firmness.
- Judging provides organisation and follow-through.

If we look at the polar opposite, ENFP, we see the contrasting preferences.

- Extraversion providing breadth and a need for human contact.
- Intuition providing vision and a grasp of possibilities.
- Feeling providing warmth and empathy.
- Perceiving providing flexibility and adaptability.

The theory predicts that the sober, sensible ISTJs will be over-represented in managerial positions – organisers love organisations! – and the statistics support this. Conversely the theory would lead us to expect that in organisations the sociable, optimistic ENFP types are usually found in the marketing department – and they are!

Finally, the type description can be uncannily accurate. If we take the short description in Jenny Rogers' manual,[4] we find:

> Thoughtful, responsible and perfectionist, ISTJs need to be in charge.
> This can be both an asset and a liability, depending on how it is linked
> to the ISTJ's skills and experience'.

Many readers will recognise a colleague – and perhaps themselves! But there is more. The MBTI can illustrate behaviour in a wide range of different contexts – leadership, team membership, ideal organisation, relationships, change. It can predict behaviour under stress. And – perhaps most usefully – it can offer a list of ways to become more effective. All these are concentrated onto a single page in the Rogers manual.

So let us look at our five scenarios and see how type might cast light on them. The first was individual:

> You have reached a decision point in your career. You have to choose
> between continuing in a specialist role, or becoming a generalist. The
> financial and promotion aspects point clearly in one direction – but
> your instincts are set in the other. How could you get a better
> understanding of your reservations in this matter?

We have seen that type descriptions can give you a very full account of your preferences for the kind of environment – for colleagues, for type of work, for leadership – that will get the best from you at work. But we can go a little further than this. The theory predicts that each type will have a dominant function – an overriding goal in life. To take our ISTJ example, type theory would predict that to be fulfilled in their work, this person would need:

> To notice and work on something useful to others, quietly, systematically, and in depth.[5]

And contrastingly, ENFPs will need 'to find lots of new and stimulating possibilities and promote new ventures'. A lens of this nature turned onto a job can be very revealing. Can the job ever satisfy the basic drive that gets you out of bed in the morning? This kind of insight can help you tell the difference between the natural prudence and caution that anyone might feel before a challenging and demanding change of direction – and a real sense that you are about to take an irreversible wrong turning.

The second was about a clash of working styles with a colleague:

> You work closely with a colleague. At first you really liked their quiet, thoughtful, undemonstrative style. But now it is beginning to drive you mad. The more you push for responses from them, the less you get. What can you do?

The more you seek a response, the less response you get. Of course there may be many reasons for this, but a good place to start is with the Extraversion/Introversion scale. Extraverts need stimulus and response from the outside world, and they formulate their thoughts by talking them over aloud. (How do I know what I think, till I see what I say?) If your preference is for Extraversion, then the Introvert's quiet internal processing of ideas – 'I think over what I'm going to say, and then I realise that having done that, there's no need to say it' – is a constant frustration to you: what are they thinking? How can I do my thinking, with nothing to respond to?

Now look at it from the Introvert's side. The more the Extravert talks, the less you can think; just when you are ready to start talking – the Extravert jumps in and fills the silence. No wonder you don't say much!

Below is a list of ways Extraverts and Introverts can communicate better. If your colleague prefers Introversion – or is using an Introvert style with you – then try:

- giving them thinking time
- giving them information in writing where possible
- waiting for a response, so that they have time to 'mull things over'
- checking things out rather than taking silence for agreement.

But communication is a two-way street. How can your quiet, reserved colleague get the best out of you? By:

- letting you talk things over
- telling you things in person, rather than in writing/by email
- giving you space for action and experiment
- allowing you to develop your thoughts as you talk, without assuming that the first thoughts should be the final conclusions.

But there is something that underlies these actions you can take. It is a change of attitude: a question, to use an earlier phrase, of 'valuing difference'. Introverts aren't just quiet extraverts; extraverts aren't just noisy introverts. Each is actually using a different process – and if you start by respecting that and allowing it to work in its way, rather than yours, you're likely to get a much better result.

Now for our third scenario. (A recent Radio Four programme claimed that one-third of complaints from patients about GPs were about 'poor communication'.)

> You are a GP. One of your recent consultations involved a very rare complaint – you have never seen one outside a textbook. You successfully identified the problem and managed, despite the patient's initial resistance, to persuade them to take appropriate action. Now, to your dismay, you hear that the patient has lodged a complaint against you! What has gone wrong?

The question of the match of communication styles between patients and GPs has been the subject of much attention in recent years. Research shows that the most common preferences in doctors are N and T (Intuition and Thinking), while the most common preferences in the population at large are Sensing and Feeling.[6] How does each group like to communicate? Research indicates that there is what we might call a 'language problem'.

People with N and T – big ideas and logic – naturally talk a particular 'language': theoretical, concise, minimal, stripped of detail, focused on the task and the problem. If they want to work with another person, they need to respect them first (if necessary by challenging them to establish that they are truly competent) – then they can build a relationship. And that is of course perfectly suited to much of the technical work of diagnosis and treatment.

But people with S and F – sometimes called 'sensible and friendly' for short – have a different communication style: practical, extended, thorough, wanting every T crossed and every I dotted, and needing to focus on the person behind the problem. For SFs, the relationship is the starting point – if they can build that, then they are willing to trust the other person's competence.

To quote a recent research study:

> If you are a patient with preferences for Sensing with Feeling (40.1% of the UK population) then you will have only a 1 in 6 chance of seeing a doctor with the same preferences. Similarly, if you are a doctor with preferences for Intuition and Thinking (31.3% of this sample) you will have only a 1 in 11 chance that your patient will be the same as you. Some adjustment on the part of one or both parties involved in the interaction is, therefore, likely to be needed if effective communication is to occur. These results may contribute, therefore, to the explanation of the number of complaints from patients about poor communication, the lack of understanding and poor compliance reported in the literature if these doctors have not learned to adjust their interaction styles to accommodate these differences.[6]

So what happened in the consulting room? Well, one hypothesis is that this is a case of a breakdown in communication between NT and SF styles. To the NT doctor, the successful outcome is a diagnosis and a treatment. To the SF patient, something has gone wrong in the relationship: perhaps they have been seen as a disease rather than as a person; they haven't been treated as a human being; they haven't been recognised as an individual. Neither side is right but something must be done to bridge the gap – and knowing something about the other person's 'language' is an essential starting point.

Our fourth scenario was about teamwork:

> You work as part of a practice team. The team has agreed its targets and objectives at the start of the year and set them out clearly in a schedule – but you seem to be the only one of your colleagues who is attending to them. In previous years your colleagues have 'got there' fine in the end, but the uncertainty, and their lack of concern, are driving you crazy. How can you and they come to some kind of agreed style?

By now you will recognise that the mismatch here is likely to be along the J/P dimension. The person with the Judging preference makes lists and plans in the expectation that they will be used as roadmaps and reference points throughout the year: that targets and objectives are not just aiming marks, but real destinations that you intend to arrive at. It looks as though they are surrounded by Perceiving types – whose attention is on the changing world around them, and whose focus is not on what was planned to be done months ago, but on what needs to be done right now. If you are indeed a J and they are indeed Ps – how can you find a way to not be driven crazy?

There is a clue in the penultimate sentence of the scenario. Your colleagues do get there in the end. Their way does work – but it fills you with anxiety (just as yours probably fill them with impatience!). If both of you are willing to respect the other's style as something that works, however strange it is to you, then here are some ways to bridge the style gap. To get the best from your Perceiving colleagues, you need to recognise that your structures and lists are not their favourite thing so you need to:

- show you are flexible
- leave space for them to surprise you
- be prepared to change your mind.

And on their side? To come half way to meet you and respect your discomfort with the unstructured and unplanned, it will probably help you greatly if they would be willing to:

- show they are organised
- give you some kind of plan or indication of how their work is developing
- allow you to complain and 'tut tut' without being too discomposed!

Our final scenario is about stress – a topic much to the fore in the medical literature.

> Mostly you handle work pressures pretty well – but sometimes you find yourself responding in a way that seems completely out of character. How can you prevent this happening again? And is there a way you and your colleagues can see it coming next time, and either guard against it, or minimise its impact?

For this topic we need to go back to the 'wrong hand' exercise. Jungian theory, and Myers Briggs likewise, emphasise that it isn't possible to be perfect – that you will always have preferences and develop aspects of yourself to different levels, so that some parts of you remain less developed than others. When you are able to use your preferred style, then work pressure is challenging and exciting. When you are pushed into using those less preferred sides, you feel stressed, and all the consequences of that come into play, just as we saw in the 'wrong hand' exercise at the start of this chapter. How the MBTI can help is to explain where your 'wrong hand' is, and how stress will affect you. If you know your four-letter type, you know what stresses that type, and you know how that type responds to stress. And if you know it, you can use that information in three ways. First, you can guard against the situations that cause you stress. Second, you can learn to recognise the symptoms, and take appropriate action. And finally, you can enlist the help of your colleagues. The more they know about your strengths and weaknesses – and vice versa – the better able they are to cover for you, to recognise what is happening to you, and to find appropriate ways of dealing with the consequences.

How do you take it forward?

- You can read more about it – there is a short reading list at the end of this chapter.
- You can arrange to take the Indicator yourself. For this you need the services of a trained and qualified MBTI practitioner, because it is a skilled process to help someone to find their type. Like an experienced tailor or dressmaker, the practitioner will help you try the suit for size and 'find the fit' – the questionnaire results are not the final arbiter, and it is a core principle of the MBTI that 'the person taking the test is the best judge of their type'. Most parts of the NHS have qualified practitioners, or the national MBTI body, the British Association for Psychological Type (www.bapt.org.uk), will provide names of practitioners in your area.
- You can go to BAPT meetings to learn more about the instrument – this chapter has only scratched the surface of its many applications. It provides sessions for qualified practitioners, but also for those with more curiosity than experience. BAPT details are given in the bibliography.
- You can explore how to get qualified – one of the joys of the Indicator is that it is possible to be qualified without being a trained psychologist. In the UK, Oxford Psychologists Press (www.opp.co.uk) has acquired a training monopoly, but in America and Australia there are a number of excellent training providers. A Google search under 'MBTI qualifying' is all you need. Surprisingly, it is cheaper to fly to Florida and qualify with CAPT (www.capt.org) than it is to qualify in the UK – and you could even take the family to Disneyworld while you're there!

References

1   Myers P, Briggs I. *Gifts Differing*. Palo Alto, CA: Consulting Psychologists Press; 1980.
2   Jung CG. *Psychological Types*. London: Routledge; 1923.
3   Jung CG. A psychological theory of types. In: *Modern Man in Search of a Soul*. London: Routledge; 1933, reprinted 1978.

4   Rogers J. *Sixteen Personality Types at Work in Organisations*. London: Management Futures Ltd; 1997.

5   Bayne R. *The Myers Briggs Type Indicator: a critical review and practical guide*. London: Chapman and Hall; 1995.

6   Clack GB. *Personality differences between doctors and their patients: implications for the teaching of communication skills*. Unpublished research; 2003.

Further reading

Further reading and information (chosen from a huge list of articles and books).

Allen, J, Brock S. *Healthcare Communication: using personality type*. London: Routledge 2001. (How MBTI can illuminate the way patients and health professionals relate to each other, well provided with examples and anecdotes.)

Allen J, Houghton A. Understanding personality type. *BMJ*.2005; **330**: 35–7.

Baron R. *What Type am I? Discover who you really are*. New York: Penguin; 1998.

British Association for Psychological Type (BAPT), 17, Royal Crescent, Cheltenham, Glos, GL50 3DA (Tel & Fax: 01242 282990). Website: www.bapt.org.uk. (BAPT is the Myers Briggs user group and provides information and events to publicise the instrument and bring users and potential users together.)

Hammer AL. *Introduction to Type and Careers*. Palo Alto, CA: Consulting Psychologists Press; 1998.

Houghton A, a series of short articles about the MBTI published in the *British Medical Journal*, which can also be found on their website, http://careerfocus.bmjjournals.com.

(2004; **329**: 191–2), Extraversion and introversion.

(2004; **329**: 202–3) How do you like to take in information?.

(2004; **329**: 213–14) How do you make decisions? Thinking and feeling.

(2004; **329**: 230–31) How do you like to live your life? Judging and perceiving.

(2004; **329**: 241–2) The whole type and how it relates to job satisfaction.

(2005; **329**: 8–9) What do type dynamics tell us about life stages and stress reactions?

(2005; **330**: 18–19) Type and teams.

Index